"In *Walking the Journey Toget* [illegible] caregiving journey and how [illegible] grace, honesty and love. She [illegible] us that we can create and experience happiness even when the odds are against us."

Jack Canfield, Co-Author of The Success Principles™

"Lorna's story will touch the heart of anyone. Especially those who are faced with caring for their loved one and wanting to do it with passion, joy and love."

Janet Bray Attwood - New York Times Bestselling Author - The Passion Test

"Heart-wrenching and heartfelt, Lorna's book is a must read for anyone needing a compassionate yet practical guide through the emotional turmoil of losing a loved one. Grieving family members and professional caregivers alike will benefit from this candid and unflinching chronicle of love and loss. I shed so many tears while reading this book, and as a person who has trouble crying, this was a rare gift. THANK YOU!!!!!!"

Karen Lewthwaite, retired women's advocate

"Cancer doesn't only affect the patient; it affects the lives of the people that surround them as well. Lorna's story provides a great first-person view into the life of a caregiver and a cancer advocate, while teaching valuable lessons she learned during her husband's fight."

Doug Ulman, three-time cancer survivor,
LIVESTRONG™ Foundation President and CEO

"Lorna Scott's *Walking the Journey Together… Alone* is an insightful and intimate look into the life of an individual, thrown into the unexpected role of a caregiver of a loved one. Her love and passion for Callum and her struggle with his fight against cancer is laid bare for the reader to share, and leads us to reassess our own priorities and lives."

Richard Smalley, Advertising Director, The Red Deer Advocate

"The journey Lorna takes us on is not only inspirational but gripping. When Lorna takes us to Scotland and recounts her *journey alone* with Cal, there wasn't enough Kleenex tissue at the computer to get me through it all.

Brad Brand, Prepress Flyer Production Supervisor, Federated Co-operatives Ltd.

"*Walking The Journey Together… Alone* is a powerful, thought-provoking love story that is a must-read for all caregivers and those soon to be in the caregiver role. Lorna Scott takes you into the hearts and minds of those affected by terminal illness and offers caring tips and reflections designed to make that final journey easier for all."

Gary Poier, Owner/Founder, Aspire Personal Achievement Inc.

"Genuine, heartfelt and impassioned. Lorna shares with us the challenges and struggles of caring for a loved one with a terminal illness. But, within that she illustrates that there can also be a deeper happiness, joy and gratitude in the most difficult of times. There are many things we can learn from her experience."

Wendy Davies, Fitness Leader and Registered Yoga Teacher

"An aspiring must read for anyone who has been or will be in the future, a caregiver for a loved one. This true life story of Callum and Lorna's love and devotion draws you quickly into their life of dreams to a life of wonder and devastation and how, as a caregiver, one can strive towards happiness."

Joan Pritchett, former caregiver

"Lorna tells her story so you can make it through your story of caregiving. Her honest reflections prompt you to tell the truth about how you feel as you care for a family member. Her book is half memoir and half journal, with space for both the reader and author to share. Lorna cares for her reader as lovingly as she cared for her husband. A wonderful resource for any family caregiver but especially for a caregiving spouse."

Denise M. Brown, Founder, CareGiving.com

"Emotional and uplifting, Lorna's story of her love for Callum and passion for caring for him is inspirational. Her message of finding peace, hope and joy is something from which we can all learn. This book is well written and Lorna is a role model for us all!"

Michael J. Hertz, Senior Vice President & Group Publisher, ALTA Newspaper Group LP

"If you've just discovered that you must step up as a caregiver for a loved one diagnosed with cancer, it may feel as though you face an unwelcome and uninvited houseguest who has full license to wreak havoc on your life. In *Walking the Journey Together… Alone,* Lorna Scott bares her soul and holds your hand, in the name of saving you unnecessary anguish. Scott's contagious optimism will help you to create unexpected moments of peace and joy. I encourage you to carry this book as a companion in your journey."

Pam Garcy, PhD, Author of The Big Book of You Don't Have To's: Free Yourself From Depression Anxiety Guilt and Shame *and author of the #1 National Bestseller* The Power of Inner Guidance: Seven Steps to Tune In and Turn On

"Lorna has written, with wit and grit, about a harrowing time. She and her husband led Cancer a merry dance for a number of years. This is a story of astonishing truth told without a whiff of self-pity. Lorna has learnt from her years as a carer and has written this book, with the help of hindsight, to give insights and reflections to other carers. The book works equally as a love story of a family coming to grips with loosing their patriarch. It is an excellent read."

Una Panting, leadership coach and consultant, The Profits of Happiness

"Lorna lovingly cared for Callum. With courage she shares her deepest emotions, the lessons she learned during their journey, and how faith and hope can help fight the odds."

Dr. Kamal Haider, oncologist, Saskatchewan Cancer Agency

Walking the Journey Together… Alone

*Finding Peace, Hope, and Joy in the Middle of the Sh***

To Betty Ann
Keep shining your bright light! :)

LORNA M. SCOTT

May you find peace, hope + joy in every day.
Lorna M. Scott
11/26/15

Book Disclaimers

Because of the dynamic nature of the Internet, any web addresses or links contained in this book may have changed since publication and no longer be valid. The views expressed in this book are solely that of the author and do not necessarily reflect that of the publisher, and the publisher hereby disclaims any responsibility for them.

The author of this book does not dispense medical advice or prescribe the use of any technique as a form of treatment for physical, emotional or medical problems without the advice of a physician, either directly or indirectly. The intent of the author is only to offer information of a general nature to help you in your quest for emotional and spiritual well-being. In the event you use any of the information in this book for yourself, which is your constitutional right, the author and the publisher assume no responsibility for your actions.

Cover and Interior Design by Stephen Ray Heppell

Edited by Kathy Sparrow

Copyediting by Jennifer Carter, Inked! Editing

Published by Accelerated Success Consulting

Most photos, except where individually acknowledged,
are by Lorna M. Scott.

The Scott Clan photo (pg 88) and Lorna & Callum back cover photo by MeKa Studios
About the Author photo (page168) by Carrie Driedger Photography

ISBN-10: 149594574X

ISBN-13: 978-1495945748

Library and Archives Canada Cataloguing in Publication

Scott, Lorna M., 1961-, author
Walking the journey together ... alone : finding peace,
hope and joy in the middle of the sh** / Lorna M. Scott.

ISBN 978-1-4959-4574-8 (pbk.)

1. Colon (Anatomy)--Cancer--Patients--Care. 2. Caregivers.
3. Caregivers--Psychology. 4. Caregivers--Services for.
5. Scott, Lorna M., 1961-. 6. Scott, Callum, 1961-2011. I. Title.

RA645.3.S36 2014 649.8 C2014-901196-2

DEDICATION

To all the caregivers who selflessly, compassionately and lovingly care for the important people in their lives. May you find your own peace, joy, and hope throughout your caregiver journey.

To my husband, Callum, who lovingly let me embrace my caregiving role, which strengthened our relationship and brought me more joy and love than I ever imagined possible. I will always love you.

CONTENTS

ACKNOWLEDGMENTS

To Callum, who had the courage and patience to stay married to me for over thirty years. He taught me many things, some I only learned after he passed away. Callum, I will always love you.

To my children, Jamie and Vanessa, and their families for the love and support during this journey. I appreciate the priority you put on being part of making your dad's last few years the best he could have. You sacrificed a lot so that we could enjoy precious family time. When I was overwhelmed by our day-to-day life you were the voices of reason that helped me take the next steps, as hard as they were. Your dad was proud of you. I am proud of you.

Thank you to my family: my mom, stepdad, mother-in-law, father-in-law, sisters, brother, brothers-in-law, sisters-in-law, nieces, and nephews. From cooking meals, doing laundry, and changing light bulbs, to gentle listening ears, laughter, and hugs, our days and my life were made better with your practical help, love, and support.

We were fortunate to build a great network of colleagues and friends as we travelled from Brandon to Medicine Hat, Red Deer, and Saskatoon. Thank you for the warm welcomes we received as we took up our new home in each city. Callum quickly built relationships with those he worked with. He was humbled and thankful for your support. Thank you to the colleagues and friends I made along the way. Many of you saw the deep pain I was in and offered your friendship and help. I really appreciated having something "normal" in my life, supported by those who understood my journey. Many of you became life-long friends.

The incredible wisdom and support Callum and I had from the great medical teams was priceless. We were always treated with respect and dignity, even when my passion for advocating for Callum surfaced. A very special thank you to Dr. K. Haider, Saskatchewan Cancer Agency. Not only did he provide the very best care for Callum, he was able to handle me. Whenever I was overwhelmed or concerned that Callum wasn't getting the best treatment, he could calm me down in only a few seconds. It takes a very special person to be able to do that. I am very grateful he was part of our journey.

Thank you to all who opened your homes to us, joined us on vacations, and were with us through the fun times and the tough times. I know you shared my pain during those six years, and continue to share my grief and pain. I wish for you to live your life to the fullest, and enjoy peace, hope, and joy along the way.

I started this book with a story. A story of life with Callum as he fought cancer. The story would not have become this book without my writing coach and editor Kathy Sparrow. Without her, I would have written a book that I think only family and friends would buy. With Kathy's wisdom, patience, and guidance I am confident I now have a best-selling book. I have deep gratitude for having her in my life.

Thank you to Stephen Ray Heppell who created the book cover and interior design of the book. He was able to take the pictures and thoughts in my head and "make me look good."

Thank you to my support team, family, and friends who have helped me in this unwanted life transition. My physical, mental, emotional, and spiritual health are much better because of you.

Many people helped us make the final years we had with Callum full of peace, hope and joy. Thank you to our family, friends, colleagues, the medical team, and others who supported us their own special way. I would like to thank each of you individually, but I have learned my memory of those years is often quite fuzzy and know I would miss some of you.

FOREWORD

Nadine Henningsen, President Canadian Caregiver Coalition

It can be challenging to care for a critically ill loved one. It can be heartbreaking as well. In this book Lorna Scott shows us that this doesn't have to be the case–not in every moment. Here, she courageously shares her journey with blunt honesty, compassion, and love about the six years she spent caring for her husband, Callum.

Family caregivers provide care and assistance for family or significant people who need support due to debilitating physical, mental, or cognitive conditions. A family caregiver's effort, understanding, and compassion enable care recipients to live with dignity and to participate more fully in society. For the eight million family caregivers in Canada, the health conditions requiring care are significant. According to Statistics Canada [2012 Portrait of Caregivers], 28 percent of caregivers provide care to a loved one with age-related conditions followed by cancer as the second most common ailment. The complex and long standing nature of these conditions are also reflected in the length and intensity of care provided by family caregivers.

The abrupt nature of the caregiver role impacts individuals of all ages, genders, and income levels. One never know when they will be called to duty. Caregivers hail from all walks of life, often undertaking caregiving responsibilities due to sudden health crises, and commonly, the onset of chronic conditions.

Family caregivers are the invisible backbone of our health care system. They often don't even recognize their vital role. They look after their family or friends because of their deep love and commitment. It is "just what they do." This is not an easy challenge. Finances can be impacted. Work affected. Dreams destroyed. Yet, many caregivers take this in stride. Somehow they make the unmanageable, manageable. Usually it is at a huge emotional and physical cost to themselves.

Lorna candidly talks about the caregiving side of the cancer story and takes us on that emotional rollercoaster of caregiving for her husband, Callum. She tells of the ups, the downs, and how two people find they are facing vastly different concerns while sharing one journey. She shows us that life can look bleak, fears can run rampant, and if you choose, you can still find peace, joy, and hope each day. Not only are we entertained by the story, Lorna gives a voice to caregivers, a helping hand to others, so that they may find their way to a more joyful and loving life. Her reflections and insights paint a picture of lessons learned all while coping with devastating news and taking care of herself. Further she shares how living life with passion and conscious intention changed her life. Her courage in sharing these vital lessons will be helpful for any caregiver.

This is not only a caregiving story. This is a story of commitment, perseverance, and the power of positive intention—a story of personal transformation. This is a story of the power of love. A story that inspires us to recognize, respect, and support the integral role of family caregivers in society.

INTRODUCTION

This book was written with you, the caregiver, in mind. During my journey through Callum's battle with cancer, I discovered many things that made our life easier and filled with joy and love. Callum and I intentionally created happy moments and lived our lives with gratitude as much as possible.

As I met other people facing similar challenges, I noticed many caregivers, especially those starting their all important caregiver role, were overwhelmed with the diagnosis, treatment, and being faced with losing someone they loved. I saw many people who were struggling to get through the day. Peace, joy, and hope were beyond their grasp.

Both Callum and I tried to help them as much as possible. We couldn't help everyone. I knew there would be a time to share my experience and help other caregivers. My passion is to help others find their way of living in peace, joy, and hope, even when their world looks bleak. *Walking the Journey Together… Alone* is my first step in helping caregivers reclaim their life, in mind, body, and soul.

Walking the Journey Together… Alone is thematic, rather than chronological. I wanted to concentrate on the lessons learned—often at various stages of the journey—rather than a day-by-day, week-by-week account of our challenges. At the end of each chapter I share my reflection on the chapter topic, which is followed by some tips and some questions for you to spend your time in reflection. This is your time. It's your opportunity to learn what may happen in your caregiver journey. I have shared my story so that you can learn from my hard knocks, avoid some of the things that didn't work so well for me, and embrace some techniques and habits that can change your life from one of drudgery and overwhelm to shared love and joy.

Being a caregiver is one of the most loving and compassionate things you can ever be, and one of the most rewarding things you can do. Typically, it comes with sacrifice. What I want most is for other caregivers not to sacrifice all of themselves while they are supporting their loved ones–both the one that is ill and family members and friends also affected by the illness.

If we had a choice, we would not be in a situation to become a caregiver. Most of us have no choice. Caregiving was one of the most rewarding experiences in my life. I hope that by sharing my experience you will also find your caregiving years to be rewarding and full of peace, joy, and hope. And while I admit that there were days when I didn't think I'd make it, I have found that there is light at the end of the tunnel, and new life to be celebrated.

Walking the Journey Together… Alone

Chapter One

The Scream

How much has to be explored and discarded before reaching the naked flesh of feeling.

~ *Claude Debussy, French composer, 1862-1918*

March 25, 2013, just after supper, I was sitting on the couch, sipping some chamomile tea with the computer in my lap. I was finishing up the last few questions for a research story about colorectal cancer patients and caregivers. The move into my new home ten days prior brought me peace and serenity I hadn't felt for a long time.

Suddenly I was taken by complete surprise. The sensation was foreign to me. The tension was building in my abdomen, becoming more intense and more fierce as the moments passed. The feeling travelled up from my stomach, through my chest, into my throat. Then I screamed. It was a loud, blood-curdling scream that originated from deep inside my body. Every cell in my body released energy. The eruption of emotion caught me off guard.

For months, both my counsellor and coach had been trying to get me to scream. I didn't understand exactly what they were getting at. I was different. I was Miss Cool, Calm, and Collected. I didn't need to scream.

I was disturbed with what was happening and moved from the living room to the kitchen. I felt better standing up. The scream escaped again. It felt undeniably liberating. I wanted more.

"Scream!" My inner voice urged me to do more. "You can do it. You need to do this. Go for it!"

My body and mind were disconnected. I played the part of an observer while this was happening. My logical self separated and was looking at a jumping bean of emotions ready to explode. I played full out with the scream. I welcomed it. I yearned for it. I wanted to get rid of that energy and make room for new vitality and opportunities. I knew this was a good thing. I screamed again.

I stood up, braced my knees, clasped my fists, closed my eyes, and screamed. And screamed. I screamed so loud I thought my neighbours would hear me and call the police. I was fearful it sounded like I was being attacked. In some ways it was an attack but it wasn't criminal. The intense emotions of grief, anger, and sadness assaulted my soul and my heart, and The Scream fought back. It was natural.

Twenty months after the death of my husband I finally started releasing the grief and the pain. I needed to release the sorrowful thoughts, the feelings of despair and sadness, and restore balance to my core essence. The world called me a widow, and that was a role I played. It was time to write a new chapter in my life.

The Scream was different from any other moments of crying and sobbing. Before The Scream, my crying sessions were about sadness, anger, frustration, and loneliness. They often came out of nowhere and frightened me. Many times I was afraid I wouldn't be able to stop crying. Up until now it was the suddenness of the tears and heartache that frightened me. The Scream was different. It was an explosion. The intensity and depth of The Scream was frightening.

I missed Callum. I started having a wonderful life and was angry and frustrated that he was not here for me to share it with him. I felt alone. He brought balance to my life, and without him I was scared of my thoughts and actions. Confidence in my abilities to make good decisions and take action was lost. I realized how much I relied on him to show me the practical side of my ideas; how much he coached me to see the details to consider when I had my big ideas; and how much I trusted him to let me go deep into my ideas, and give gentle guidance so that I stayed away from huge mistakes. He also let me make mistakes so I learned my lessons. He'd give me just enough rope to let me find my own way without hanging myself. It became a struggle to discover and develop those qualities on my own—or to find someone who could fill that void. My head was overrun with the negative thoughts of "people will think I am crazy." Callum loved me for me. He believed in me. I didn't have to explain "me." After thirty-four years of being together that made sense.

In the twenty months since Callum passed away, I was busy. Busy trying to move on. Busy trying to figure out my place in the world. Busy trying to sort out my idea of a normal life for a widow. Busy trying to figure out how to be a mom and a grandma, without having a dad and a granddad by my side. Busy trying to find the place to spread my roots.

Just plain busy.

And most of all, I was busy running from the grief and running away from me … coming to know me again—perhaps for the first time in my life.

I dealt with the grief by trying to fill myself up, create something new. The problem was I hadn't let go of the past. Callum was not physically here and he continued to be an integral and embedded part of me. I still spoke "we" instead of "I." I often wondered, "What would Callum do, say, or think?" There were even times when I had the thought, "I can't do that. He doesn't like it."

The fall after he passed away, I went to Manitoba to celebrate the twenty-fifth anniversary of his brother and sister-in-law, Alan and Dorothy. Alan took me to play a round of golf. I was low on golf balls and was deciding which ones to buy. Alan picked up a yellow one.

"Here, this one would be good for you," he said.

"I can't buy a yellow one," I politely stated. "Callum hated coloured golf balls."

"He's not here anymore," he reminded me. "You get to choose what you want."

It was true. I could choose what I wanted. I just didn't know how.

These messages, feelings, and thoughts from our relationship as husband and wife were ingrained into my being. For six years I set aside anything to do with me. I immersed myself into doing everything possible to make sure Callum had the best treatment and care he needed to beat cancer. Habits were formed, taking over my own self-identity. I stuffed away my own feelings and fears. I had to do something with them. Scream. That was what The Scream was about. That's how this was different. I was setting "me" free.

I had intense feelings. Feelings of anger. Anger that Callum was gone. Anger that he didn't go to the doctor sooner. Anger that my mother-in-law's doctor never told her to make sure her boys got screened early. Especially that. It would have saved his life. Anger that his dad went through the same thing over seven years later. I thought everyone in the family had taken action to get screened. I didn't know how the message didn't get to Walter or his doctor. His son was diagnosed with Stage 3C colorectal cancer, and died from it. I won't ever understand why my father-in-law, at seventy-four years old, never had a colonoscopy and no doctor made sure he had one. That situation reactivated anger and frustration hidden in my body and mind. All of it provided additional fuel for The Scream.

Feelings of sadness were part of the mix as well. I missed my husband. I missed not having someone with whom to share my thoughts, excitements, and disappointments. I missed his cooking—oh yes, his cooking. I missed his hugs, kisses, and gentle touch. The way he could look at me, smile, and instantly warm my heart. I was sad that my two grandchildren would grow up without their granddad. I felt sad knowing that when our son chooses to have a family, they will not have the pleasure of knowing the dad that Jamie respected so much. I was heartbroken that life had forever changed.

These were some of the things buried deep inside me. These are things I had held onto for years, things that encapsulated me. It was time to release the energy needed to keep them, and give them a place of honour. It was time to turn them around and create strength and hope. It was time to build a new foundation and create a cornerstone for the future. It was time to release, to let go, to no longer be anchored by the weight of grief.

All of these thoughts and feelings were buried deep inside for years. There was no coincidence The Scream happened ten days after I moved into the house I had built. It was full of my own personal touch. I felt grounded and safe. I finally felt like I was home. Peaceful and comfortable, it was the perfect environment to start the release process. I was ready to take on challenges, opportunities, and dive into the excitement of my future. I had to let go of energy that paralyzed me so that I could refuel myself with gratitude and optimism for the future.

I managed about five minutes of screaming before I was utterly exhausted. I could feel the energy release from my body. The feeling was so good I wanted more. I wanted to get rid of this energy. I wanted to make space for the future. I wanted to make space for me.

The future became filled with relief and hope. There was relief in letting go of these emotions and habits that had filled my life over the past few years. Emotions and habits that were buried in my role of caregiver. There was relief from no longer having to carry the weight of caring for Callum on my shoulders. There was relief. Good old-fashioned relief. When I closed my eyes, I could see the relief pouring out of my body, opening up room for hope and the future. I could feel the rush of energy fill my body, mind and soul. I could see things in a positive light. I was gaining my identity back. I was a step closer to knowing "me" again.

Feelings are much like waves, we can't stop them from coming but we can choose which one to surf.

~ Jonatan Mårtensson

REFLECTION

In looking back over my years as a caregiver, I realize that I could have probably avoided The Scream, if I had made time to honour my own needs, wants, and emotions. Instead, I gave all of me away—to Callum, to my children, and even to our extended family and friends.

TIPS

1. Screaming can release a lot of pent up energy. Practice screaming as soon as you can—and do it often—whenever you feel the urge. Find a safe place away from others when you do this. It can help to go somewhere that noise will cover the scream; for example, sit in your car with the radio turned up loud.

2. If you don't find screaming helpful, do something else to release the energy. For example, stomp your feet, go for a walk/run, write in a journal about your feelings. The important thing is that it is something that helps you get in touch with the deep, hidden feelings of grief.
3. Punch a pillow to start the flow of emotion that will help release a scream.

TIME FOR YOUR REFLECTION

1. What do you think and feel when you are encouraged to scream?
2. What have you been frustrated or angry about? How have you dealt with those feelings? Did it help?
3. If you are able to give yourself permission to scream, what did your scream feel like? What did it sound like?

Chapter Two

Emotional Derailment

If you're going through hell, keep going.

~ Winston Churchill, British politician and Prime Minister

The ticking of the clock reminded me how long I had been waiting. I looked at the suitcases sitting side by side at the door. It was the last weekend in September, and Callum and I were heading to Medicine Hat for a weekend of golf. My heart pounded with excitement as I closed my eyes and looked forward to the fun we were going have with family and friends.

I'd been waiting for over two hours for Callum to come home from his appointment with the specialist. I was sitting on the couch when I heard the door open, and without looking up, said, "I hope you had something really good to read!"

The silence was deafening. I put my feet on the floor, first one, then the other, stood up, and turned to face him. His brow was all wrinkled, his eyes had a piercing sadness to them, and the overall look of fear told me something was serious. The look on his face scared the hell out of me. I could tell he was trying to be strong, but his voice, softly trembling, gave it all away, "I have cancer."

In a sudden swoosh, all strength left my body and I crumpled back down on the couch.

In the blink of an eye, my life changed forever. It wasn't the first time we faced cancer in our family. Our great-niece had a bone marrow transplant a week earlier in her fight with leukemia. Callum's mom was diagnosed with colon cancer in 1984. It didn't matter what I thought I already knew, when I heard those words spoken, it felt like a thousand razor blades ripping at my heart. I was paralyzed by the shock.

This was the first time the shield of armour came to protect my mind and my heart. It provided protection until I had time to process this unbelievable news. To say I was stunned is an understatement. I managed to stand up again, and went over to Callum to give him a hug. I expected to start crying, but even when I tried, there were no tears. Everything in my body had shut down.

It was Friday night and we could do nothing about the cancer, so we continued our trip to Medicine Hat. Through most of the three and a half hour trip I felt like I was in a soupy fog. Occasionally, the reality set in. I'm living in a nightmare. As soon as I had that thought, my brain put up the protective shield of armour. At some intellectual level, I knew what Callum said to me. Cancer. He said cancer. I heard the words. They just weren't sinking in.

Callum diligently focused on the stretch of highway in front of us. It was his distraction from this cruel news. Eerily, it was a metaphor for the rest of our lives. We were in the dark, heading out on the road of cancer treatment, not knowing where it would go or where it would end. Finally, the shield started to come down, and my brain began filtering the news. A full two hours later, the tears started trickling down my face. First one, then another, then streams and streams of tears. My husband has cancer. My heart had awakened to the reality. My husband has cancer. My mind raced, thinking about the dire possibilities. My husband has cancer. I wonder if he will soon die. I had to find out more about what this meant and what we would have to deal with. I was scared for Callum and what this meant for him. I was petrified what it meant for me.

I wondered if I had what it would take to make it on my own. I had never lived alone. I left my parents' home when I married Callum. I never had to be self-sufficient. He was the family provider and the last few years were focused on him and his career. Whenever we moved, I accepted whatever job suited me at the time. The truth was that financially I would be looked after whether he continued to work, or if he died. I wasn't sure how I would make it through the "in between." There could be loss of income, increased drug costs, travel expenses. The fear overcame me. My brain sucked every ounce of energy to process the information, protect my emotions, and formulate the next steps.

"Are we saying anything to anybody this weekend?" I asked. I had never had so much trouble getting words from my head to my mouth.

"Only the kids for now. There's no point in saying anything until we know more about what is going on," Callum said, his voice void of any expression.

We decided to only worry about what was in our control that weekend. Thank goodness he was Mr. Practical. I would have been blurting the news out to anyone we met, asking what they knew about colorectal cancer and treatment.

For the rest of the trip, we sat in deafening silence. This was not the trip I was happily looking forward to only a few hours earlier. We were thrown into a world full of uncertainty, trepidation, and fear. Everything we dreamed about for our future came to a screeching halt. This was definitely one of life's defining moments. I thought I knew what it might be like to be personally touched by cancer. I quickly realized I knew nothing. That scared the hell out of me.

I thought back to the times I heard about someone having cancer. I remembered having a "punched in the gut" feeling for a few minutes and feeling sad for the family. The picture in my mind was of someone looking thin, grey, and with no hair. My life carried on. I thought of them very little after first hearing the news. When I would later hear that they beat it, I would imagine they were back in perfect health. When I would hear they succumbed to it, I would feel immense sadness. Not once did I ever remember thinking about the "in between." That was where the real story of cancer lived.

Callum must have been overfilled with emotion. Even though we agreed to tell only our children, as soon as we walked into my sister's house, he blurted out the news. I stood there in shock, not used to him acting this way. He usually kept it together. After letting it all out, he calmed down and decided to call his parents. These conversations helped him discharge some emotion and gain some strength before we told Jamie and Vanessa, our son and daughter, later that weekend. We both knew that telling our children would be the hardest of all.

A few fun days of golf did little to release the fear of the unknown. There was a lot to deal with and to think about. When we returned home, I joined Callum and took two days off work to regroup. It's not like I could have really focused or concentrated on anything anyway. I'd have been totally useless at work. I used this time to be quiet, just "be" with him, and wait for the next steps.

Waiting was not my strong suit. I liked to be in action. Yet my body felt like it was full of lead, and I couldn't move if the house were on fire. The only thing that relaxed me was cuddling with Callum. His gentle touch was soothing and helped me believe that everything was going to be all right. We spent our regroup time talking about the fear we had about what lay ahead. We waited for the doctor's office to call with appointments — ones that I had hoped would move us out of this waiting game and put this behind us. While we waited, we cuddled, rested, and watched a few funny movies. Laughter was the best medicine, particularly as the game turned to one of "hurry up and wait." I used to equate the word cancer with the word crisis and thought we should be rushing to see doctors and have more tests done. I wanted things to happen fast so we could get this over with. Let's just get it done! It didn't work that way.

After what seemed like an eternity, Callum got a call with times for appointments on the following day. On the schedule was the colonoscopy, chest x-rays, and blood work. Another thing we learned about the medical system was that things were always open to change at the last minute. We thought he would only be going for a colonoscopy. The game plan changed without us knowing it. However, we didn't really care about the extra time. Our philosophy and commitment was to do whatever it took to get rid of the cancer.

Tuesday was a very scary day. It felt like the rest of our lives were hanging by a thread, and whatever happened would forever set the course for our future. On top of our minds were the results of the colonoscopy. Callum was brought back into the holding area after his the procedure, and I had never seen him so nervous. He was very solemn, anxious, and couldn't carry on a full conversation. I tried hard to make him laugh or smile. Nothing seemed to work. When I looked at him, my heart broke as I wondered what he must be feeling. He was so young, only forty-four years old.

Dr. Simmonds came into the room. Another man joined him a few minutes later.

"Mr. Scott," Dr. Simmonds said. "As you know, there is a tumour in your rectum. The good news is I didn't find any other ones during the colonoscopy. There were only a couple of polyps, and I removed them. I took two pieces of tissue for the biopsy, which should be back in a week to ten days. You will need surgery. I am in the process of retiring and asked another surgeon, Dr. Muirhead, to join us today."

Callum politely greeted Dr. Muirhead, and then timidly said, "OK. What does that mean now?"

I was still green in this medical world and I sat there and said nothing. I wrote some notes, hoping to not miss anything important. The shield of armour went back up.

"What this means is that we will do surgery to remove the tumour, and I will make a referral to the cancer clinic. Usually, they recommend a combination of chemotherapy and radiation before surgery to shrink the tumour. It gives a better chance of success," he said.

Callum's voice trembled as he asked yet another brave question, "What does this mean for a prognosis?"

"I would say a fifty-fifty chance for five-year survival," Dr. Simmonds replied.

My stomach flipped. The shield came down. It wasn't strong enough to protect me from everything—particularly what I needed to hear. I needed to know what we were dealing with. I knew he needed me to be in this, and not always hide behind an invisible wall. I looked at Callum and was surprised to see he looked relieved. After the doctors left, he finally spoke.

"Well, that was better than I expected," he said, with a lot more confidence in his voice.

"What? This isn't good news!" I exclaimed.

"I thought I was going to be told I had only three months to live and to get my affairs in order," he explained.

It was all about perspective and ours was vastly different. Before the colonoscopy, I believed he would be like his mom, beat cancer and go back to living a normal life. This was far more critical than I had previously thought. I now understood why he looked so serious and scared earlier.

Five weeks later we were making our way around the Tom Baker Cancer Clinic in Calgary. It was nerve-racking to say the least. There were so many people there. Some looked no different than we did. Some were blunt reminders of why we were there. Bald heads, arms that looked like they were only skin and bones, skin that was grey or greenish in colour. Cancer. Right there, in front of our faces, was evidence of the future.

We met with a medical oncologist, Dr. Sasha Lupichuk, and the radiation oncologist, Dr. Chan. By the end of the second day, we had the treatment plan. Callum would have five weeks of a combination of chemotherapy and radiation. The chemotherapy would be administered continuously through an IV using a PICC line. The chemotherapy drugs were in a bottle, nicknamed a "baby bottle" because of its size and shape. The bottle would be attached to him for the five weeks, with the exception of when he would get a new one each week. He would have daily radiation treatments five times a week. It was made clear to us that this meant he needed to stay in Calgary from Monday to Friday. This intrusion into our lives was made so much easier when Callum's family friends, Stuart and Ann, opened up their home to us for those five weeks. Their hospitality and support made a big difference and helped us get through the toughest time in our life.

I used to work with people in crisis and thought I knew the physical effects a crisis brought onto a body. It was only during this time I truly understood how suddenly the physical and emotional effects could be felt. Entering the "cancer zone" was more than about treating the physical disease. Emotions, many of them I've never felt before, came exploding to the surface. Conflicting emotions rose up every day, and I was reminded of a book, *Double Dip Feelings* by Barbara S. Cain, MSW, which I frequently referred to when I worked at the YWCA Westman Women's Shelter in Brandon, Manitoba. Cain explained how we could feel two opposite emotions at the same time. This was a perfect description of what it was like feeling fear and sadness about a cancer diagnosis, and at the same time, feeling happy it wasn't worse. The body and mind had ways, like the shield of armour, to lock away emotions to preserve much needed energy for dealing with the shock. Otherwise, the emotions would have brought me to my knees and rendered me useless. Even when my world was falling apart, the mundane everyday tasks still needed to be done. I still had to work.

The shield had a counterpart that also kicked into play—my inner robot. It was the only way things got done. The robot took on the important tasks of going to work and the details of building a house. Many of the things that were extremely important before now seemed inconsequential. It was hard to concentrate on paint colours for the new house when I was faced with losing my husband. That's where the robot came in handy. The choices were made.

Many times I listened to people at work complain about someone putting a toy back in the wrong place, and I wanted to yell, "Who cares? Is anyone dying over this?" Our lives were already different, and treatment hadn't even started. There were so many unknowns about what would happen with the cancer treatment. The robot kept me on course. It seemed like the only way to survive.

Callum got through the five weeks of treatment with only a few bumps in the road. He was given time for the radiation to continue to work and for him to recover from the pre-surgery treatment. Everything lined up well for the February 6, 2006 surgery to remove the tumour.

Filled with conflicting feelings Vanessa, Jamie, Mary, Walter, and I visited with Callum before he was taken to the operating room. I looked forward to the great news that the cancer was contained and Callum would be cancer-free. Yet I was afraid that something would go wrong in the surgery, or they would find something unexpected. I pushed the fear aside and focused on believing everything would go as expected, if not better.

After the surgery I saw Dr. Muirhead in the hall and asked him about the surgery.

"The surgery was a success," he explained. "We were able to remove the tumour and the margins look good. We won't know absolutely for sure until the biopsy results are back though."

"That's great news!" I said, relieved. "What about the colostomy?"

"Unfortunately, the tumour was too low and I had to remove the whole rectum. He will have a permanent colostomy. We had been prepared that the whole rectum may need to be removed. While the permanent colostomy was not the outcome we hoped for, it was a small price to pay to be cancer free.

A few days later the biopsy results confirmed that the margins were good, which meant that all the cancer they could see was removed. It also confirmed that four of ten lymph nodes were positive for cancer cells. It wasn't the worst of news, but it wasn't good news. The perspective on the prognosis varied, and the best he was given was a 60 percent chance of a five-year survival. For now, he was cancer free. That was the important thing. There was no room for any doubt in our minds that Callum would be cancer free for a lot longer than five years.

There were days I wanted to run and hide from this new reality. I questioned my strength to see this through. I looked at my husband, who looked perfectly healthy on the outside. It made no sense to me that he could be so sick. There were moments I felt sorry for myself. As if that helped anything. It was easy to do, though. I would see the pity in people's eyes and I heard it in their voices. This startled me back to the reality of the gravity of the situation. Then I knew I had to pull up my big girl panties and carry on. I wanted to yell at the top of my lungs that Callum was not one of "those" cancer patients. He was different! We didn't need pity. He was a survivor and would always be one. Even when I was overcome with fear, I put a smile on my face and bravely exclaimed there was nothing to worry about. I had to believe it. I had to proclaim it. If I kept saying it out loud, it must come true.

Sometimes at night the feelings would sneak out. While lying in bed, I put my head on Callum's shoulder. When my tears touched his skin, he gave me a squeeze, and soon I felt his tears as they rolled down his cheeks and landed on my face. There were no words. Only tears. Together in silence we let the sadness sneak out, one tear at a time. I was afraid that if I ever really started crying I would never stop. I honestly wondered if it was possible to run out of tears.

When I heard of a fifty-fifty chance of survival, I was pretty devastated. One of the key things I learned was that Callum and I often had different thoughts, perspectives, and reactions to what was happening. The difference in perspective did nothing to change our combined determination and laser focus on beating this disease. I saw that we were in this together, and that it would be different for each of us. I had to find a way to cope with being intimately affected by the diagnosis even though I was not the one with cancer. The disease attacks one body, and infiltrates the hearts and minds of many, many others.

Life is not about how fast you run or how high you climb but how well you bounce.

~Vivian Komori, founding partner of The Broad Perspective Network and CEO of Lomoris Connections, Inc.

REFLECTION

I had a sneak peak at the shield of armour the day Callum was diagnosed. I tried to figure out what was happening, and what was ahead of us. I've heard it said that most people's biggest fear is being told they have cancer. Mine was that my loved one would die. There are no words to really describe how I felt, or what happened to my body and mind when Callum told me he had cancer. I felt the shield of armour protect me from the depth of my emotions. Thank goodness. It was uncomfortable and a little clunky at times. The shield created a wall between the real world and me. It stopped the bad news from attacking my heart and let it more gently settle in, a little at a time. It gave me strength to get through the day without sad and angry emotions exploding out of me at will. I was glad it was there. I was grateful for the robot as well. It kept me on track so life didn't completely crumble around me.

TIPS

1. Research and learn as much as you can about the cancer type and treatment (or other chronic illness, disease, or disability). Sometimes the patient likes to do this. If this is the case for you, ask how you can support them.
2. Accept that some days will be tougher than others. The feelings of overwhelm can come out of nowhere. Plan in advance by having some things ready to comfort you. A good book, inspirational readings, or audio, talking with a good friend, taking a ten-minute (or longer) walk are all good things to keep in mind.

3. Find someone to talk to about what is happening. Talk as much as you can with your loved one so you have a good understanding of how each of you are feeling, and what you need in order to cope with this kind of news.

TIME FOR YOUR REFLECTION

1. How have things changed in your life since you first heard your loved one has a chronic or terminal illness or disease?
2. Are there any questions about the disease or treatment that you would still like answers for? Who do you need to ask?
3. In what ways does the cancer diagnosis affect you differently from your loved one? What are your fears? How do you communicate them?

Chapter Three

Control Freak

We don't see things as they are, we see them as we are.

~ Anaïs Nin. American author

It was inevitable. I came face to face with the control freak in me. I liked to pride myself on being rational and too evolved to be a control freak. There was evidence to the contrary. The control freak served me well. I also bore the scars from when the "control freak goes bad."

From start to finish, during the journey of Callum fighting cancer, I struggled with what I could control and when to throw my hands in the air and cry "uncle." Sometimes my control was necessary; sometimes I fooled myself into thinking I had control; and sometimes, many things were out of my control. Most often it was the latter.

I had been a control freak most of my life. Callum understood this and loved me anyway. I ignored the fact that even though I presented a great argument, rationalization, or justification, I still couldn't control what someone else did. My temper tantrums, coercing, and silent treatments were not strong enough weapons to make someone else change what they thought or did. The control freak thought otherwise.

Even before he was diagnosed with cancer, I tried to control his ideas about going to see a doctor. Vanessa told us that her doctor recommended

Callum be screened for cancer ten years earlier than the age his mother was diagnosed, and he was already nine years past that point.

I pushed and prodded Callum. He described it as nagging and said, "I feel fine. Only sick people need to see a doctor."

I tried everything from gentle nudging, ignoring the situation, to pulling out my bitch card. It was all met with silence or outright resistance. I was a slow learner.

"Did you call a doctor?" I would ask.

"No, I didn't," he said harshly.

"When are you going to call?" I asked sharply.

He raised his voice. "I'll do it when I am good and ready!"

He had total opposition to do what was best for him. Our conversations would end in a huff. This cycle went on for a few months and, after a while, we skipped the niceties and would go straight from "did you call a doctor?" to snapping at each other. Eventually I figured out I was not going to win this battle. I could only hope that he would soon see a doctor, and that there were no bad surprises. I thought back to his mother's bout with cancer eighteen years earlier. She was lucky, caught it early, and has been cancer free ever since. I had no reason to think anything was wrong with Callum. He seemed healthy enough and had no complaints. I would still feel relieved if he would see a doctor and get everything checked out. Men. They hate doctors. I didn't want to admit that this was totally in his control. I was not going to change his mind.

A year later, after moving to Red Deer, the cycle repeated itself. After twenty-five years of marriage, I still hadn't learned that when it came to Callum, he was really the one in control. He finally admitted he had been having some rectal bleeding for a couple of months. I didn't want to jump to conclusions about the rectal bleeding and knew that forty-four year old men, and women, often had hemorrhoids or other minor issues that caused rectal bleeding. If I were a betting person, I would be betting on the hemorrhoids. Yet there was still no need to ignore the sign. He had decided to see a doctor at a walk-in clinic. I was nervous about what a walk-in doctor would be able to do for him. There was no choice. The only way you could get a family doctor in Red Deer was to go to a clinic and hope the doctor you saw had room to take on new patients.

Callum was fortunate. He saw Dr. Grundling, who had room in his practice. I was very grateful for that.

Callum was referred to a specialist to find out more about what was causing the bleeding. Weeks went by and we heard nothing from the specialist's office. I got increasingly frustrated with him. He was far too patient about waiting to hear about the referral. More time went by without hearing anything and I tried to ask him about it. He was aggravated with me. I didn't know what tactics to take without the conversation ending in a fight.

"Some days there is bleeding and some days there isn't," he snarled, flashing me a look meant to stop a charging bull. "You are too impatient," he challenged.

He believed he would hear from the specialist's office when they had an appointment time booked for him. I tried not to harass him about it, but every once in a while, I was at the end of my rope and the words blurted out of my mouth. In the end, the fight just wasn't worth it. In the name of peace, I backed off and left him in control.

I got more and more aggravated about waiting so long. Eventually, Callum lost his patience and checked to find out what was happening with the referral. For more than three weeks, he called the specialist's office and left messages that were never returned. When he finally got a live voice on the phone, he was told the referral never made it to the specialist's office. To add insult to injury, he was also told the specialist was going on sabbatical and not accepting any referrals. He was back to square one. I was livid. My control freak wanted blood. I was infuriated at the time that was lost. I had no idea what was wrong with Callum. I knew it was getting worse and I wanted it fixed. No more monkeying around. I came face to face again with the control freak, when there was no control to be had. Its presence was with me throughout this journey, from his diagnosis to his death.

Seizing Control

There were hard lessons to learn. The medical system generally worked well. I could understand that it was an overloaded system full of paper trails and sometimes things would hit a snag. I learned that ultimately it is up to the patient to take 100% responsibility and make sure that their files, referrals, tests, and test results get to everyone who needs them. That's the best way to let the control freak reign.

I still wish I had found a way to exert more control before he was diagnosed. I could have taken more responsibility for that, and I dropped the ball. He would have been diagnosed sooner and could have started cancer treatment a year earlier. I wish I had dug in my heels about the initial referral to a specialist. Knowing I was right only fuelled the control freak's desire to have power over the situation.

I decided then and there to do whatever it took to get the satisfaction of being in control. And I did it by taking notes at doctor's visits. Before each appointment, I reviewed the notes from the previous visit to see if there was any follow up needed. I always had my notebook and pen with me. When we were in the appointment, the physical act of writing down information kept my emotions in check and became the record of what the mind had difficulty processing at that moment. I used the notes to settle arguments between Callum and me about what the doctor said and/or did. In my self-righteousness I believed I was armed with information, and could outsmart any doctor or medical professional. I was the broker of all information about Callum and the many things he endured. I was the top dog. That was really what it was about. It was about my control, and keeping control, in a situation that was truly out of my control. I really fooled myself.

The control freak thought she had it all figured out. Much to my dismay, the note taking was another area where I couldn't always be in control. In early 2008, when Callum was referred to a surgeon to remove the two spots in his lung, I did my research and came up with a list of questions. I couldn't go with him and was apprehensive about teaching him to ask questions and take notes. He better remember the list of questions I gave him! We were so different when it came to dealing with medical professionals. He was such a model patient and listened to what the doctor said without clarifying or asking questions. I questioned everything the doctors said and made sure I found out they were on track with how they treated him. He did ask the questions and take good notes. I was happy.

I couldn't control the cancer. I couldn't control what the doctors would do. I could control my questions and my notes. And I could control the knowledge I had about what was coming around the corner. I found some salvation by doing a plethora of research.

Knowledge was power. The control freak feasted on research. I dove into researching everything I could about diagnosis, staging, treatment, and outcomes. Once I knew what I was dealing with, I could meet it head on. Anticipation and the unknown were not my friends.

The research was scary and depressing. In the initial stage of the diagnosis and treatment, I found a lot of information on staging cancer. I was not surprised to find out it was Stage 3C, which meant that the tumour had broken through the bowel wall, but not into the fatty layer outside the bowel wall. The initial outlook was not positive, with only about one third of patients with Stage 3C colorectal cancer living more than five years. This was not enough to beat us down. Our positive outlook was, "Well, Callum may as well be in that one third!"

Other times, the research I found was very positive and relieved my fear and anxiety. I found out that the protocol of having combined radiation and chemotherapy before initial surgery came out of research done by Dr. Chan, the radiation oncologist who treated Callum. It was much easier to trust that he was getting the best possible care when a researcher of the new treatment method was treating him! He was lucky, not once, but twice.

In 2008, when the cancer spread to his brain, I spent hours and hours on the Internet doing research. There was little information to be found on brain metastases. It was not usual for colorectal cancer to spread to the brain. Callum had already proved himself to be an unusual patient. It was no surprise he continued down that path.

He was referred to a neurosurgeon, Dr. Fourney. I did my due diligence to make sure I approved of Callum being treated by him. I was a lot more confident about insisting on changing doctors if there was reason to believe he was not receiving proper treatment. I was impressed by what I found about Dr. Fourney. He completed his neuro-oncology internship at M.D. Anderson Cancer Center, one of the top cancer centres in the world. He also worked in Germany on research for Gamma Knife Radiosurgery treatment of brain tumours and other diseases of the brain. He was cutting edge when it came to this treatment.

Gamma Knife Radiosurgery is a non-invasive brain radiation treatment and is very successful at treating brain tumours and giving a longer life to patients. It was no wonder that Dr. Fourney made the referral to Dr. Michael West, head of the Gamma Knife Radiosurgery department in Winnipeg, Manitoba. Research showed that he was instrumental in bringing the Gamma Knife Radiosurgery technology to Canada, and Winnipeg was the first place in Canada to offer this treatment.

Knowing that these doctors were the best of the best, and Callum would be in good hands, comforted us. The control freak was pacified.

Relinquishing Control

There were times that cancer and its circumstances controlled me. Believe me, I didn't want to admit this, but it was true. I was not sure which was the scarier thought, that something could control me, or that I actually admitted there was something I couldn't control.

After his initial diagnosis, I was committed to supporting Callum through thick and thin. I requested time off from work to stay in Calgary with him when he had pre-surgery chemo/radiation treatments. My mind had been in a fog since we found out he had cancer and I couldn't imagine not being with him through treatment, especially when he had to be away from home five days a week. I had started the job four months earlier and had little vacation time to use. My options were limited and I was determined to do whatever was necessary to be with Callum for those five weeks.

One day, I was sitting in my office when the head of the organization showed up at the door. I explained to her what was happening with Callum and why I needed the time off. She seemed open to the idea and told me to officially put the request in writing and send it to her. I felt quite hopeful that I had explained the situation well and expected the approval would be a formality.

I was appalled when I got the reply to my request. I received approval to take the four days vacation I earned so far. For the remainder of the four weeks, I was expected to work part time. The suggested schedule was to take Callum into Calgary Sunday night, go back to Red Deer to work Monday and Tuesday, return to Calgary Tuesday night and Wednesday, back to work Thursday, then drive back to Calgary Thursday night or Friday morning to pick up Callum. If I didn't want to drive, or the roads were bad because of winter weather, they suggested I take an express bus into Calgary. It was clear that I was expected to work three days a week. I did not find this acceptable in any way, shape, or form.

I felt bullied. There was no compassion, empathy, or understanding of my situation. When backed into a corner, I felt the "fight or flight" syndrome run through my veins. With a strong urge to just up and leave, I decided instead to fight for what I needed. I didn't want to play the sick card, but felt forced to. I went to my doctor and she, somewhat reluctantly, gave me a note for a week off sick. I took it to my employer who, reluctantly, accepted it. I was flabbergasted that an organization which provided services to people of all ages had such little compassion for their employees. We had just moved to Red Deer, had little support, and any friends we had were acquaintances from work. I had no idea what side effects he would have to this treatment and was extremely frightened to be that far away from him. The radiation oncologist insisted that Callum remain in Calgary from Monday to Friday, and it was at least a one and one-half hour drive from our home to the hospital or to where Callum was staying. These facts did not in any way change the decision. Basically I was told to suck it up or leave. I could not understand why she wasn't more compassionate about how devastating and frightening all of this was to us. I managed to get the doctor to sign a sick note for an additional week off work. That took care of the first three weeks. It was the best I could manage in a situation that controlled me.

Even with the disagreement and stress about my time off, I wanted to keep my immediate supervisor up to date on how things were going. She was very supportive and I was grateful for her understanding and support. Part way through the third week, I started to believe I was feeling and doing better. I was more comfortable with the routine of daily visits to the hospital and knowing that Callum's parents were there to help. I considered returning to work part time. I received an email from my supervisor that said that I was required to return to work at least half time or else I faced being laid off. As I stared at the computer screen reading the email, the tears immediately welled up in my eyes and started to trickle down my cheeks. I felt a knot start to grow in my stomach and thought I was going to throw up. The tears ran down my cheeks and my heart raced. I was suddenly flooded with emotions and realized if looking at words on a computer screen could invoke such an intense emotional response, I was not ready to return to work. Their command to return to work was not negotiable. I was very distressed and wanted to just say, "Piss on it. I quit!"

Callum was the king of logic and convinced me that it was not worth losing a job over a few days of time off. He assured me that he would be well cared for by his parents and our friends. I gave in and realized that if I wanted to keep this job, I had no more control of my time off. The only real control I had was whether or not I wanted to keep the job. It was such an oxymoron to me that the agency that prided itself on supporting families did not support me. They expected that I could physically and emotionally continue to provide good service to the families I worked with. When I did return to work, I provided little support for them when I was an emotional wreck myself. They deserved more than I could give. I played the game and showed up, physically, anyway. My mind was 150 kilometres away, in Calgary, with Callum. So be it. There was one thing I was firm about, though. I would not work for that organization any longer than I had to. I discovered one of my deep core values, and sought out employment opportunities that gave me the flexibility needed to be able to give Callum all the support he needed, and that I wanted to give him. Compassion, empathy, and importance of family would be things I looked for as I went forward in any job positions. My days with that organization were numbered.

When the control freak reared its ugly head, I was frequently met with frustration and disappointment. I lost time and energy trying to create the world I wanted and avoiding reality. I couldn't control him, and still I kept trying. I wanted him under my wing and I needed to know his every move, twinge, and pain. He had other plans.

Callum and his brother Alan had a special bond. It was very important to Callum that he support his brother and insisted he be at Alan's farewell dinner as President of the Canadian Professional Golf Association. The fact that he had major surgery five weeks earlier and just finished his first round of chemotherapy didn't phase him. Normally, I would have gone with him and wished with all my might that I could. I had no vacation time left. I used all of it for his medical appointments, surgery, and treatment. Enter the control freak.

I had become so intertwined with him and his health that I was sick with worry about whether he was healthy enough to make the trip. I worried that his immune system was too low and he would pick up some deadly virus on the plane. I worried that his incisions were not completely healed and he would get an infection. I worried that no one would watch him close enough to make sure he didn't take any chances, and they would miss key signs that he was getting sick and needed to see a doctor. I ranted and I raved. There was no stopping him.

It all worked out fine and he came home feeling better than before he left. Callum–one. Control Freak–zero. I continued to grasp onto whatever control I could find. Callum filtered through this insistent need of mine. He gave me lots of leeway up to the point where he would obstinately disagree with me. I'd be reminded of who controlled him. He did–it was him, and only him, who would make these decisions.

Much to my dismay, more ranting and raving, we went through two more rounds in this bout of going away without me. I wanted to trust him, I really did. But I knew he would not complain to anyone if he was not feeling well. He would push himself. I worried about whether he would get enough rest. I feared he would get sick. Callum–two, Control Freak–zero. There was no way I could control him.

The unpredictable aspects of cancer and cancer treatment often took control of me. On a nice sunny Saturday in June 2008, I poured myself a cup of freshly brewed coffee. I took a deep breath, smiled, and sighed at the thought of finally having a nice quiet and relaxing day to hang around the house. The last few weeks had been busy with moving into our new house, Callum starting chemotherapy, the diagnosis of brain metastases, and having company. We deserved a quiet weekend to ourselves and basked in sweet peace on this beautiful day.

The serenity I felt was sharply cut when I heard Callum exclaim, "I think we need to go to the hospital."

I turned around and saw him walking down the hallway from our bedroom, holding up his left arm. It was swollen and very red and purple. He was right. He needed to go to the hospital. I was normally filled with compassion and ready to do anything for him. That day, my first thought was, "Really? Now what?" My perfect day was ruined.

I was irritated. I had the day planned, and looked forward to some peace and relaxation together, and instead we were going to the hospital. The frustration lead to moments of anger at how this damn disease managed to stick its butt into the best of moments.

We found out Callum had a blood clot that went from his wrist all the way up to his shoulder. He had the PICC line removed. He was given heparin (an anticoagulant, or blood thinner) to inject each day at home until he saw his regular oncologist for further treatment options. Six hours later we returned home. I had to have a careful watch over him. There was a small chance that the blood clot would break off and go into his lung, causing a pulmonary embolism, and a high risk of causing death. This would not be a relaxing weekend. Another day lost to the beast of cancer treatment.

Sunday started off as a quiet, albeit a relaxing, day. Just as Callum was ready to give himself the injection of heparin, the phone rang and it was the oncologist on call who wanted to speak to him. I handed the phone to him and they had a discussion about the anti-coagulant. Callum finished the phone call and told me that Dr. Arnold, the oncologist on call, said that he needed to take the heparin because of the blood clots and risk of a pulmonary embolism. The risk with taking the heparin was that it could cause the brain tumours to bleed, causing a stroke. As Dr. Arnold so eloquently said, he was between a rock and a hard place. Her recommendation was to continue with the heparin, and if any symptoms of stroke showed up, he was to get to the hospital immediately. He was to go to the hospital if he had any trouble breathing. That would be a sign of a pulmonary embolism and require immediate medical attention. Not one, but both days of the weekend were ruined. My dream of a relaxing weekend was quickly replaced with worry. There was no relaxing to be had when every minute I wondered if he would have a stroke or quit breathing.

I was dazed with this news. I didn't have a lot of room left in my brain for more problems. I desperately wanted to put Callum in a bubble so nothing more would happen to him. I felt like I should sit and stare at him, watching his every breath. Waiting, wondering when something worse would happen. Even as a caregiver, I was being controlled by this wretched disease and treatment side effects. Throughout the day my mind wandered, pondering how much longer his body could go on, and how much more it could take before it gave in and stopped. I felt battered, being slammed over and over again by the insidious cancer. I wanted to stay positive but so much had gone wrong in the last few weeks that I knew to be prepared for the worst that could happen. When I allowed those thoughts to escape, I felt like I betrayed Callum. He fought so hard—how could I think it's not enough? I tried to push those thoughts away, but the flood of thoughts and feelings took over my body and mind. He rested during the day while the battle between hope and reality raged inside of me.

I took a stack of frozen burgers out of the freezer and started to separate them with a table knife. They were really frozen together so I found a sharper knife. Callum might not feel like eating. Is there any use in cooking supper?

The sharp pain in my hand was the first indication that something had gone horribly wrong. My mind was snapped back to the present. I looked down to see the blood running from my hand. I had not been paying attention to what I was doing and the knife slipped from the burgers and into the fleshy side of the palm of my hand. There was sharp pain at the beginning, and then it quickly left. I looked at my hand and saw it was quite a deep cut. As quietly as possible I snuck into our bathroom, found some gauze and wrapped up my hand, trying to be careful that the bandage wasn't noticeable. I didn't want Callum to know about this. I was embarrassed and didn't need him worrying about me or being mad that I wasn't paying attention to what I was doing. I returned to making supper and noticed new spots of blood on the counter. I took a look at the bandage and there was no blood there. I looked at the back of my hand and noticed a small cut. The knife had actually \gone all the way through my hand. How did I not see that the first time?

Thankfully it looked like I didn't do any serious damage to my hand. I snuck back into the bedroom to redo the bandage and as I looked at it, I realized that I should go to the hospital for stitches. Now I was between a "rock and a hard place." I needed medical attention, but would live whether or not I got it. Callum wasn't in immediate need of medical attention, but if something changed, it would happen quickly and time was of the essence. I didn't feel comfortable leaving him alone. In fact, I was petrified to leave him alone. I put my own needs on hold, and decided to go to a doctor the next day if I needed stitches. I managed. It was just a cut. Cancer had taken control of where my needs were unmet. My control freak lost again.

Two major control issues came into play. Both had a direct affect on me and our relationship. He had ultimate control in both instances—one had to do with him continuing to work, the other had to do with his decision about his treatment plan. The control freak didn't give a damn and I went head to head with Callum over both. I charged into the fray even harder. I knew what I wanted and I strived to get it.

Callum insisted on working even after being diagnosed with two brain tumours and told he likely had much less than a year to live. I knew if I had the chance to choose how I would spend my last few months on earth it sure as hell wouldn't be at work. For the life of me I couldn't understand why he was so damn different. There were so many things I wanted for him, for us, before he died. This was our only shot at retirement together. My heart ached as I watched precious hour after precious hour slowly fade away, never to be recaptured. I was determined to change his mind. I asked a social worker to ask Dr. Ahmad, the oncologist, to tell Callum he didn't have long to live and should not be working. He always did what his doctor told him to do.

At the September 2008 appointment with Dr. Ahmad, two months after the diagnosis of the brain tumours, we were taken into a room with soft pink coloured walls, comfortable chairs, plants, and soft lighting. This was quite a contrast to the regular clinic room that had the bright lights, an exam table, sink, and small desk for the doctor. The cancer centre was a very busy place and they used every nook and cranny. Dr. Ahmad and his nurse Margie came into the room.

"Mr. Scott," Dr. Ahmad said, "Do you realize how sick you are?"

The light bulb went on in my head. We were in the calm room. We were going to have one of those tough conversations. This was not going to be a pleasant visit.

Dr. Ahmad gently, calmly, and bluntly talked with Callum about the seriousness and reality of the cancer and it spreading to the lungs and the brain.

When asked for an updated life expectancy, Dr. Ahmad said, "in this situation you can expect six months and, if you are lucky, maybe up to a year."

I wasn't sure which part of my body felt the sting first, my stomach, brain, or my heart. Six months, even a year, didn't seem very long. Suddenly, the once devastating life expectancy of eighteen to twenty-four months "before brain tumour" seemed a blessing. It was amazing at how quickly my perspective changed. Dr. Ahmad continued and, not so gently, suggested that maybe leaving work would be a good idea.

Callum sat tall in his chair.

"I understand the prognosis. I am not ready to give up fighting and I am not ready to leave work."

When we got home, he told me that if he left work, he would feel that he had given in and given up, and he was not ready to do that. That was a point where I wondered when my opinion would matter. Both of us were fighting for his life. Callum and I shared a goal of making the rest of his life the best it could possibly be. We disagreed on what that meant and were miles apart on what to do next. My picture was of a few short months of retirement and, damn it, I wanted some fun. I wanted us to do the things Callum had always wanted to do and see. Until then we hadn't talked about these things and suddenly I realized I didn't know what he wanted to do before he died. I imagined there were some important things, and I wouldn't have thought work was one of them. I felt forced into doing what he wanted with no regard to how I felt or what I wanted. Or what his family wanted. Vanessa had said for months that she wanted to spend time with her Dad when he was still feeling well and able to do things with her. She told me she hoped he would take the time to be able to enjoy visiting with her, Stuart, and Jamie. His parents and brothers lived 1,100 kilometres away. I was sure they would like to have some quality time with him. If he continued to work, I couldn't see how we would find the time for all these visits. Callum was the one with cancer. He was not the only one whose life was changing because of it.

This was his fight and the cancer treatment was his decision and choice regardless of how it intimately affected others. He might not have felt the need to be closer to family or to have any kind of a bucket list. He might not have needed to hold onto anything, and everything he could. My heart was heavy with the thought of regrets should he continue to work. There was no way to change his mind. He continued to work and I continued to wish he didn't. Callum–three. Control Freak–zero.

The other major issue the control freak jumped into was Callum's decision to continue chemotherapy treatment with only months left to live. He wouldn't give in. He wanted to make sure he had every possible opportunity to stay alive long enough for a new treatment option or clinical trial. I wrestled with the contradiction between knowing there was little to no hope for a cure or any options to extend life, and fighting tooth and nail to hang on, just in case a miracle happened. The discourse came with how each of us dealt with it.

I wanted to enjoy our time together. I wanted us to enjoy time with family and friends. I didn't want to be a slave to chemotherapy treatments, doctor visits, and ongoing tests. It wasn't the cancer that was making him feel physically unwell—it was the treatments. Callum's goal was to live as long as he possibly could. No regrets, we agreed on that. I struggled to make sense of why he would want to spend the rest of his life getting sick from chemotherapy. I felt so passionate about this that I wanted to grab him and shake him until he regained some sense. It was his body, his mind, and his choice. I was not in control. This was a pivotal moment in time for me, to have someone else determine whether or not I could have what I so deeply desired. I wondered if this could be, even a little bit, compared to how Callum felt knowing that this disease was slowly sucking the life out of him, even with his deep desire to live. Our future was slipping through our fingers. There was no victor in this round.

I learned to be careful what you wish for, and I was thankful for unanswered prayers. I had a deep desire for Callum to discontinue treatment after finding out he had two brain metastases. I truly believed we had only a few months, at best, left together. I wanted to stop the rest of the world and concentrate solely on our relationships and everything Callum wanted to do before he died. I wanted treatment to end in September 2008. Thankfully he was persistent, in fact, down right stubborn. He did not want to give in. I realize now that had he given in, I would have been right, we would have had only a few months together. This is a case where I was thrilled to say I was wrong and he was right. I profoundly believed that continuing with treatment was instrumental in prolonging his life by nearly three years.

Ironically, my goals were also reached. We enjoyed many good times together and with family and friends. He did get to check off some of his bucket list, like owning a Porsche Boxster, seeing AC/DC and U2 in concert, and taking our children to Scotland to meet ninety-year old Nana Campbell and other family. The lesson here was to have faith that the cancer patient knows their body, their mind, and their will to live. Reality is that living with a terminal illness did not end in a win-win situation. I have come to better understand that when a person is dying they hang on to as much control as they possibly can. What they choose for treatment is their decision, and the rest of us must adjust. Callum knew what he wanted to do, he knew he wanted to keep fighting and there would be a purpose for that. I adjusted my opinions, learned to trust him, and unconditionally moved forward with him.

This happened a few times over the six years. For much of this, his journey really was a "we" journey. These were two of the times that we had opposite opinions and saw things completely different. I was so very thankful that I eventually had the wisdom to let him lead on these issues. By submitting to his desires, I came out a winner.

Diverting the Control Freak

Constantly fighting for control was exhausting. When there was a bombardment of bad news, I went dizzy into a downward spiral. There had to be a better way. There had to be something I could throw myself into, something that would keep me busy. I was a fixer and a doer. I didn't give in. If I couldn't control Callum's cancer, I had to find a way to make a difference for others.

In April 2008, shortly after we found out that he had terminal cancer, he was loaned the book, It's Not About the Bike by Lance Armstrong. Callum refused to read the book so I decided to read it. It was my first in-depth introduction to Lance Armstrong and his LIVESTRONG™ Foundation. His reputation as a cyclist was later in disrepute, and I wished he had decided earlier to come clean on using drugs when he was cycling. As I read the book I kept thinking that Lance Armstrong was an arrogant man. There were many instances when reading the book that I didn't particularly like him. I also learned to admire the fight and positive attitude he had when battling testicular cancer. I was truly grateful he decided to form the LIVESTRONG™ Foundation (www.livestrong.org). The Foundation helps many people get through their time with cancer in as positive and healthy a way as possible. Lance Armstrong was able to leverage his celebrity status to help millions of cancer survivors around the world. That was no small feat.

I was so inspired by the organization that I realized I had found the positive outlet for the control freak. I joined the LIVESTRONG™ Grassroots Global Community in their fight against cancer. It was that moment I decided if I had no choice and was going to be part of the world of cancer, I wanted to make a difference. I wanted to become an advocate and bring awareness of local cancer issues to my community. I became a LIVESTRONG™ Foundation volunteer and created the Saskatoon Supporting LIVESTRONG™ Community Cancer Corporation (SSLCCC).

The control freak's appetite was satisfied and happy about focusing on something other than work and cancer treatment. I recruited to the group some of Callum's staff and a couple of people who worked in my office building. With a few other volunteers, our group had about five active people. I was flying now and could hardly wait until Saskatoon heard our message. Immediately, we got into action and participated in a Global Conversation on Cancer. With some emphatic cajoling, I managed to convince the group to agree to bring The Giant Colon Tour to Saskatoon to celebrate LIVESTRONG™ Day on October 2nd. Okay, I say emphatic cajoling. The control freak bordered on bullying!

I talked with the representative at the Colorectal Cancer Association of Canada about The Giant Colon Tour and knew this was a great opportunity to make a huge impact in Saskatoon. The CCAC rented to people the forty-foot long, eight-foot high, inflatable colon and there was reams of education provided with it. It was a very unique way of drawing people into learning more about colorectal cancer, and just what the control freak ordered. This would make a difference. People had to know how deadly colorectal cancer was, and how preventable it could be. They would learn, even if I had to shove it down their throats. The plan was in place and with fundraising and promotion underway, the group worked hard through the summer to make LIVESTRONG™ Day 2009 an unforgettable day in Saskatoon. Callum loved having my attention put somewhere else. He got a well-deserved break from the control freak.

LIVESTRONG™ served up another positive outlet to make a difference. I applied to be a delegate at the LIVESTRONG™ Foundation Global Cancer Summit in Dublin, Ireland in August 2009. I used The Giant Colon Tour as the required community project that would demonstrate an impact of cancer awareness in our community. I fed my need for control, and all the energy it brought, for a higher purpose. I gathered facts, created a project outline, proposed outcomes, and submitted the application. I was excited by the opportunity and also had some trepidation about what would happen if I were selected. I wanted Callum to come with me and for us to enjoy a vacation in Ireland. He wasn't fond of the idea. I refused to give in to his objections. The dark side of the control freak returned.

I emphatically decided he would come with me and he would have a good time. He put up a valiant fight to stay home but it didn't matter to me. I unilaterally decided he would come and booked our flights. He'd have flipped if he had ever found out how much his flight cost. In my opinion, there was no price too high for our enjoyment. Now he had no choice. He had to come with me.

The last week in August 2009 we flew to Dublin. It felt like a dream come true. Less than nine months earlier I hardly knew what LIVESTRONG™ was or what it meant. There I was in Dublin, a delegate to their Global Cancer Summit. This was the embodiment of inspiration and awe.

We settled into our hotel and got some sleep. The next day Callum and I took a walk to the location of the Summit so I knew where I was going in the morning. It was a typical summer day in Dublin. The sky was overcast with a hint of rain. Well, drizzle. There was just enough to drag along the umbrella, but not enough to get it wet. Along the walk, we passed some pubs and bistros that looked quite interesting. We passed a small corner grocery store where we could get some snacks or medications. A few more steps down the sidewalk, I looked across the street and saw the large, white building.

"This is it," I thought to myself.

My heart started beating faster. It was unbelievable I was there! We crossed the street and noticed the large white and yellow LIVESTRONG™ banners. Words of hope, encouragement, and survivorship were written on the sidewalk in bright yellow chalk. The excitement and anticipation of what was to come ran like a freight train through my veins. I was sincerely amazed, and the summit had yet to begin.

Over the next three days I joined five hundred delegates and listened to expert panel discussions, participated in group brainstorming and sharing, and learned how to effectively communicate our message when we returned home. The meal times provided ample opportunities for learning. One day, I sat at the table with a doctor who was part of pioneering the United Nations campaign to address the AIDS epidemic and was doing a similar thing for cancer control. Another day, I spoke with a pediatrician who worked in Peru and was trying to set up a way to use computer and teleconference technology to better treat children living in remote areas of Peru. I was humbled by the brilliance with which I was surrounded. Many times in the day I gave myself a pinch to remind me this was real.

The greatest take away from the Summit was that anyone, and everyone, could make a difference. From the grassroots level in our own backyards, to international doctors and lobbyists who worked tirelessly to provide dignity and respect to all who were fighting cancer, I learned each one of us could make a difference. I finally found there was something I could control. Through education, awareness, and advocacy I could have an impact in my own community. I thanked the control freak for seeing the opportunity to be part of a higher good.

As they say, you can lead a horse to water, but you can't make him drink. Callum did not have a good time. He stayed in the hotel room for the first two days, only leaving the room for meals. He told me he just couldn't get over the jet lag, was tired, and not feeling well. I convinced myself he was having a temper tantrum because he had to spend time alone. I did all this for him and he didn't even appreciate or try to enjoy it.

I had put the blinders on and later realized that I insisted on putting my needs ahead of his, and tried to make him enjoy what I thought he should enjoy. I forgot, or refused to acknowledge, that he was not me. I would be excited to go exploring on my own. Callum was not very adventurous on his own. Maybe he really did have trouble getting over the jet lag. I couldn't help but wonder how quickly he would have recovered if we were here for a newspaper convention or on a trip with his friends. Callum and Control Freak were tied on this one.

October 2, 2009 was LIVESTRONG™ Day around the world and the public launch of Saskatoon Supporting LIVESTRONG™ Community Cancer Corporation. This was the first time The Giant Colon Tour was held in Saskatoon and Midtown Plaza, and the downtown mall was the scene for this exciting day. The forty-foot long, eight foot high, inflatable pink colon was standing by, waiting for the crowds to go through it and learn about diseases of the colon, polyps, and colon cancer. I had invited government officials and sponsors to join us in our launch. It was a big hit. Over 1,800 people went through the Giant Colon that day. I had helped make an impact in our community.

Eventually you realize that not all opposing viewpoints come from people who oppose you.

~ Robert Brault, writer & blogger, U.S.A.

REFLECTION

For nearly six years I fooled myself into thinking I had to control so much of the medical information. I kept many detailed notes, appointment schedules, test results, and doctor's visits. I collected so much information it filled two binders! I pause and wonder how many trees I have killed and how many hours I have spent collecting all this data. I look back and see many hours I could have used to look after myself better.

I could have spent the time getting a massage, reading, or working out. I could have spent the time making healthier meals and freezing them for the busy days. I could have meditated. I could have talked to a friend, gone to a movie, or talked more with Callum. I could have looked within to see what I needed, to find ways to cope better. It just seemed so important to have the information, carefully organized into tabs in the binder. It was busy work, and had little to do with anything that had happened, or would happen. I had given up on looking after me. The outcome of this was that I stayed overweight, went on anti-depressants, and lost my sense of self. I had clenched my jaw so much that it took a year after Callum passed away to totally release. The clenching caused cracks in some of my teeth and some have broken. There were many long-term effects of not caring for myself. The lesson here was that the one thing I could have controlled was my self-care. I probably would have been better prepared to take care of those around me had I done so.

TIPS

1. Taking notes at doctor visits is a great way to keep track of important information. It has been suggested that we often only really comprehend about 30% of what is said at an appointment with an oncologist. Writing down the information can help you focus in a different way and give you time later to re-read and process it. It is a way of finding out all you need to know and not having to emotionally deal with it at the same time.
2. Writing or journaling can give you the opportunity to express your feelings, worries, and hopes. This can be done privately. Some people like to express things more publicly, perhaps in a blog. This can be helpful when wanting to keep others updated about what's going on, and it often helps others going through similar circumstances. I did this for over three years.
   Visit: www.calupdate.blogspot.ca
3. Post the Serenity Prayer (or something similar) where you will see it often. It is a good reminder to think about what is actually in your control.

TIME FOR YOUR REFLECTION

1. What areas of your life, especially your caregiving life, are you trying to control? Are you really in control of these things?
2. How are you hurting yourself by trying to be in control of the uncontrollable?
3. What would it feel like to give up control?

Chapter Four

The Worst That Could Happen

Perseverance is not a long race; it is many short races one after another.

~ Walter Elliott, Scottish politician

For over two years we enjoyed a well-deserved reprieve from the chronic stress. Regular follow-up appointments gave us the opportunity to celebrate each time Callum was spared treatment. Each victory and celebration built up our strength and we were lulled into a sense of security that all would be fine. Even when there was a possibility the cancer had spread to a lung, the optimism of the oncologist, coupled with the fact that he had already faced cancer head on, left us believing this would only be a little inconvenience in our lives. Surgery and chemotherapy, no big deal. Been there, done that. Once again it was "let's get it done" and move on with our lives.

The wheels of the medical system started turning and soon everything was in place in Saskatoon for biopsy surgery to take place on April 14, 2008. I had a lot of fear and anxiety about the surgery, and I was ecstatic that now we were one step closer to Callum being cured.

I was convinced that there was no need to dust off my protective shield of armour. I was so strong now and everything about our experience with the Saskatoon medical system had been impressive. I liked the convenience of the pre-admission clinic at the hospital and having everything done in three or four hours.

Callum and I spent Wednesday, April 9th at the hospital for the pre-op admission tests. The last one was checked off the list and we got ready to leave. The clerk stopped us to let us know the surgeon wanted a CT scan before surgery and it was scheduled for the next day. I was a little miffed at the inconvenience of having to be back at the hospital the next day, and at the same time impressed with the thoroughness of the surgeon.

Thursday, we returned to the hospital for the CT scan, the last test before surgery. Callum checked in at admitting and headed over to the CT/X-ray department, then down another hallway to the CT scan area. He drank his usual goop and the technician inserted the IV line for the contrast dye used in the scan. I patiently waited, as usual, for everything to be done. It's not like I was able to help in any way, but Callum appreciated me being there for the support. I was happy to give it to him. This was lung surgery and I could understand that the doctor wanted the most up-to-date information. She had left no stone unturned which relieved my fears and anxiety about her ability to look after him. Before we could go home, there was one more stop to make. We stopped to see Dr. Kennedy to go over the CT scan results. We walked into the waiting room to see six people waiting to see a doctor. We found a spot on one of the bright orange couches, picked up some reading material, and waited.

One by one, each person went into a room to see a doctor, came out, and left. Soon we were the only ones in the waiting room. Callum looked at his watch, looked up at the clock on the wall, put a scowl on his face and muttered to himself. It was after 4:30 p.m. We had been at the hospital over three hours. He hated waiting! He had only one more day at work to get things in place before he'd be away recovering from surgery. This was cutting into his preparation time.

"Callum Scott." Finally, he was called into Dr. Kennedy's office.

Dr. Kennedy's office was small. There was a chair next to the doctor's desk and the spare chair was behind the door. Dr. Kennedy came into the office, shut the door, and we introduced ourselves. She had met Callum once before. This was the first time I had met her. I was anxious waiting for her to come into the room. Going through this serious surgery with new doctors in a new medical system made me nervous. However, once I met her, I could tell Dr. Kennedy had a down to earth personality and she quickly put me at ease. I knew he would be in good hands.

"I asked for the CT scan today to confirm what I thought I saw in the PET scan," she began.

I expected to hear that maybe the spots had grown and that surgery might take longer or be more complicated.

"Mr. Scott, the CT scan shows multiple spots in both lungs," she paused. "There is no point in doing surgery. I am so sorry."

I was caught off guard. I didn't expect bad news and didn't pack my shield of armour. I thought I heard the surgeon say she wasn't doing surgery. I thought I heard her say there was no point, and that there were multiple spots in both lungs. I didn't comprehend the gravity of the latest news. Well, spots in both lungs. Can't they just take out the spots and leave the lungs?

I mustered up the courage to quietly ask, "How many spots?"

"There were eleven in the left lung," she said.

I wasn't sure I wanted the answer, but asked anyway, "And the right?"

Her voice was quiet and soft, "We quit counting."

This was the worst thing that could happen.

Last time we found out about the worst thing that could happen, I remembered feeling like I was punched in the stomach. Not this time. Today, I felt like I was hit with a steel girder. I was amazed at how calm Callum seemed to be. Usually, I am practically and emotionally prepared for whatever could happen at a doctor appointment. There was no denying I was not prepared for this. For the past twenty-six months, we held tightly onto the hope there would still be a cure. "Two or three small spots in the lungs," we were told. "Take them out and there was still a good chance to be cured." We were always given words of hope.

Those were magical words. It didn't matter now. I sat in the chair, unable to speak. My body and mind were numb. The shield of armour was now in place. I looked at Callum and the doctor, and realized that my husband was going to die. Soon. I didn't know how I managed to keep breathing with this feeling of a twenty-ton weight on my chest. I squinted my eyes, trying to make sense of what Dr. Kennedy said. My heart raced. I wanted to say something, but the words in my head weren't making any sense. Even after all the hours I spent learning more about the disease, treatment, and progression of the disease, I never expected this. I tried to make some sense of what was happening. How can there be that many spots? I wondered. There were only two in January. Well, there had been three and two joined together, but there was certainly not eleven! My hand shook as I picked up my pen to write down this very important information. This couldn't be happening. I was not prepared.

"What are the next steps?" Callum asked.

"I will contact the Cancer Centre and let them know the situation and see if they can get you in to see an oncologist soon," Dr. Kennedy replied. "The oncologist might want a biopsy of the lungs before he plans treatment. Given the progression of the disease it's possible he won't need it and will just move forward with chemotherapy. So, I can give you a choice to think about. The time is booked in the operating room anyway. I can do the biopsy on Monday and then you would have it done if the oncologist needs it. Or you can wait until you see the oncologist, and if he needs the biopsy we can schedule it then."

"If we wait until we see the oncologist, and he needs the biopsy, how long before surgery would be done?" I asked.

"We could likely schedule it about two weeks after the oncologist's request," she answered.

This was all too scary.

Dr. Kennedy continued, "Another thing to consider is that if you have the surgery, it means you likely can't start chemo for five to six weeks."

The words seemed like they were in slow motion, and I used every bit of energy in my brain to attempt to capture and understand this conversation.

"So," says Callum. "I can have the surgery, which I might not really need, possibly delay chemo five to six weeks. Or not have the surgery, find out at the oncologist's visit that it's needed, wait two weeks for surgery and then another five to six weeks before I start chemo. Or, there is a possibility

I won't even need the surgery. Is there any way to find out if an oncologist would go ahead with treatment without a confirmed biopsy from surgery?"

"I'm not sure," she said. "I can try to find out for you, though." And then she paused again. "To delay treatment four to six weeks will have little change in the outcome."

Callum took a minute to collect his thoughts.

"Well, if I don't need the surgery I would prefer to not have it. But I don't want to delay treatment, either. Hopefully we can get an oncologist to give us an answer."

Dr. Kennedy said she would do her best to find out some information, and we had until early Monday morning to make a final decision.

"Thank you for all of your help, Dr. Kennedy," Callum said as he rose and shook her hand. I managed to get out of my chair and shake her hand.

I remembered looking at her and seeing her mouth move as she was talking, but not one word entered my brain. My body was numb. I wondered if she noticed the fear in my eyes. As we left the office, paralysis slowly took over my body and my thoughts. My thoughts froze and my legs were like lead pipes, making each step a challenge.

We left the Outpatient Department in silence. An hour earlier we were counting down the hours to Callum being cured. Abruptly there was no cure. There was no hope. We were quickly thrown back in time to those feelings of the initial diagnosis. It was time to resurrect those shields of armour that protected the deep and intense emotions that were starting to surface. I remembered those inner robots that helped us get through the practical matters that needed attention without being completely immersed in the emotions. My world had changed forever. Again. This was the worst that could happen.

We continued through the tunnel, down the stairs, and got into our car in the parking lot.

"What now?" I asked Callum.

"I don't know," he said, very somberly.

I looked at him and saw that his eyes were glazed over and there was no emotion showing on his face. I knew from past experience this was his "thinking" face. There were so many things to consider about the next step and it felt like there was no clear-cut win. It was a long, silent ride home.

Much of the strength we built up over the past two years was suddenly being called in to battle. It was like déjà vu all over again. New city, new jobs, new house, new cancer. We pulled ourselves together and knew we would deal with whatever was slammed our way. It wouldn't be easy. We were tough. Callum was really tough.

This experience taught me a lot. I learned to never expect a normal doctor visit. Many times I psyched myself up to hear bad news, and was joyously elated when the news was good. Other times I was ready for the "same old, same old," only to get slammed by bad news. This time, everything pointed towards a real chance at a cure. More than ever before in the journey I was slammed with the unexpected. That was why the automatic functions of the inner robot took over. The day-to day things still needed to get done. Phone calls needed to be made or returned and doctor appointments had to be kept. Something deep inside moved my body to complete necessary tasks while protecting my heart from the hurt and devastation.

With no answer from any oncologist on whether or not a lung biopsy was needed to create a treatment plan, Callum made the courageous decision to have the biopsy surgery as planned. The surgery went well, and it was confirmed that the lung lesions were from the metastasized colorectal cancer. That step was done. The next step was the oncologist appointment.

I had never felt so nervous before meeting a doctor. I was more nervous than when I met Callum's first oncologist. I wanted to believe that Dr. Kennedy was wrong. I wanted to believe there was a mistake in the CT scan results. I wanted to wake up from this nightmare and find out that he could still be cured. I desperately wanted some hope.

The oncologist, Dr. Ahmad, introduced himself and started to tell us about the spread of cancer to the lungs. He got right down to business.

I picked up my pen and notebook and started writing notes when he looked me square in the eye and firmly said, "Mrs. Scott, you don't need to take notes. I will write everything down for you."

This had never happened before. I was now terrified of what he was going to say.

Dr. Ahmad reviewed what we already knew. There was no cure. All that could be done was to try and slow down the disease.

"Are you interested in hearing about the average life expectancy at this stage? Some people like to know, others don't," Dr. Ahmad asked.

He spoke with confidence, softness, and compassion. His caring eyes looked directly at Callum while he waited for an answer.

"I want to know what I am dealing with," he insisted.

Dr. Ahmad continued, "The average life expectancy is eighteen to twenty-four months. It varies depending on the patient."

Two years. That was not a long time. Callum took the news of eighteen months to two years life expectancy as a challenge he had to face. He was very competitive and had always been a high achiever. He was determined to show the doctors he was not average. In this new life, we took on whatever was necessary for him to outlive any expectations, and maybe even live long enough to have a chance for a new treatment, maybe a cure.

The rules of engagement had changed, and Callum was ready. I was ready. This didn't mean there weren't bad days. In fact, many moments were similar those first few days after the initial diagnosis. I was afraid, hopeful, and determined. Realistic and optimistic. Those were two very opposite outlooks to have, yet equally important. This was the worst that can happen. I vowed to get through it.

Cancer didn't discriminate. It didn't care if you had no rectum and had a colostomy. It didn't care if it had spread to both lungs and terrifyingly took the wind out of your sails. It grew and grew. There was no fairness. There was no reason. It just was.

We were now in a new "cancer zone." Callum started chemotherapy two days before we moved into our new home in Saskatoon. My shield of armour was in place to protect me from my emotions and the inner robot looked after the practical things that had to be done. There was no time or energy for emotion.

I was at my wit's end with all the things that needed to be done and how much time it was taking me to deal with moving into our new house and with Callum and his treatment. It didn't take long for him to start getting mouth sores. He was incredibly crabby. Everything was about him. How he felt. What treatment was coming up. What I had to do for him. And the house. And work. This was a marathon, not a sprint, and I really needed to get re-energized. I finally came to terms with the fact that our future was uncertain and would be lived around chemotherapy and doctors' appointments. I kept waiting for the down time when I could start to get some rest, relaxation, and build up those strength credits. I was drained. *Please, let me find strength.*

In June 2008, Callum came home from work with a severe headache, and I couldn't help but be concerned. He said there was a headache flu going around the office, and insisted I not worry. I gave in and decided to believe he could have a flu, just like anyone.

The severe headache didn't subside and Callum missed another two days of work. I'd had enough. I called Dr. Ahmad. He ordered a CT scan of the head. He told us it was only a precaution and he was not worried, so we didn't need to be. He prescribed some Tylenol 3 that was to help with the pain, but it mainly let Callum sleep. My concern grew when the pain refused to subside. Callum continued to reassure me it was just the flu, just like the people at work.

Friday was the appointment for the CT scan, and by then we believed it was a waste of time. Callum was starting to feel a bit better and I was thankful and happy he was over the flu. I had to admit I was disappointed we missed many of the usual good days. This was supposed to be our good weekend and he still wasn't feeling back to his regular self. The next chemo treatment was just around the corner. Headache or not, there was not much that would keep him from his chemo treatments. They were his last hope.

I was relieved when Callum returned to work, and I could get back into my office to try to figure out what I had to get done. I tried to stay on top of it all, but so much had happened in the previous month. Being in the office gave me a little glimpse of normalcy and was a welcome reprieve.

The reprieve was short. After we got home from work that day there was a message from Dr. Ahmad. Callum called him back.

"Mr. Scott, I am sorry to tell you that the CT scan shows two spots in the brain, one about four mm and the other one is about one mm. I still don't think they are cancer. I have ordered an MRI for tomorrow so we can find out for sure what they are," Dr. Ahmad said.

On such short notice we were lucky to be able to shift our work schedules for the next day. The normalcy of going to the office was short lived.

I tried my best to not worry about the spots. Dr. Ahmad said they weren't anything large enough that would have caused the headache last week, and colorectal cancer rarely spread to the brain. I could still hold on to hope that it was the flu last week and the small spots showing up on the brain were something other than cancer.

It was chemo week and suffering from the side effects of the chemo started early this time. On Thursday, Callum stayed home from work. I was so thankful for such a flexible job so that on days like this I could work from home. The peace of the afternoon was sharply interrupted by a ringing phone.

I looked at the call display and saw it was someone from the cancer centre calling.

"Hello," I answered.

"Hello, this is Dr. Ahmad, can I speak to Mr. Scott, please?" I knew this was not good news. We didn't get phone calls from the doctor unless there was a problem.

"He's resting right now. Can I help you?" I hesitantly ask.

"I would really like to speak with him," he insisted.

"I'll see if he's awake," I replied.

I went into the bedroom and found Callum lying awake on the bed. I told him Dr. Ahmad wanted to speak with him. Callum picked up the extension phone by his side of the bed. I stood next to the bed, beside him, and used the other handset to listen to what Dr. Ahmad had to say.

"Mr. Scott. I am sorry to tell you that the spots on the brain are cancer. I will send a referral to a neurosurgeon," Dr. Ahmad explained. "If you haven't heard anything by the end of next week call Margie, my nurse. It looks like surgery should likely be an option, but the neurosurgeon will decide that. There will likely be radiation after surgery. We will have to stop chemo two weeks prior to surgery. I'm not sure what will be done if surgery is not an option."

I looked at Callum. I saw him first start to scowl and then bite his lower lip. I saw the disappointment in his eyes. I stood next to him in disbelief and resignation, feeling like I'd just been punched in the gut. For a few days, I had grasped tight onto hope there was no more cancer. My world was shattered. We had to find more hope. Hope was the thing to get me through this. This was the worst that could happen.

I didn't want to believe that anything else could happen. I hadn't even got used to the fact that Callum was on chemotherapy to prolong his life, and I had to deal with the news of two brain tumours. Life wasn't fair and we found that out fast. I was emotionally and physically battered.

I had never been more scared. I was on pins and needles wondering what would happen next. I couldn't imagine there was anything worse that could happen and knew I had to entertain the possibility there was more to come. This was a mental battlefield.

The next five months were filled with medical appointments, tests, and treatment. The ongoing medical issues seemed to have hit their limit. My focus and concentration turned to keeping track of the busy treatment schedule and caring for Callum on his sick days. Somehow, I managed to maintain some semblance of a work life. Perhaps that was the distraction that kept me sane and hopeful.

There was no disputing the disease was going to progress—and it did right into the bones.

The lesion found on his femur in 2010 pretty much disintegrated the end of the bone near his knee. There was bone rubbing on bone causing intense nerve pain. The disease weakened the bones so he could no longer put weight on that leg. It would be crutches for him forever. A round of low dose radiation helped alleviate some of the pain. The weakened and damaged bone caused a lot of mobility issues. The constant and intense pain affected every minute of his life.

One of the palliative home care nurses recommended seeing the pain specialist. Dr. Haider, the oncologist, had been working with us to manage the pain and agreed it was time to talk to the pain specialist. This was a vital step in helping Callum get back some quality of life. And for me to get back some sanity.

By the end of the year I learned how to manage his pain using narcotic painkillers. Maybe we would get back a normal kind of life. He was still trying to be tough and not take as many as prescribed. My job was to convince him that he experienced breakthrough pain because he didn't want to give in and take the medication regularly. I couldn't blame him. The medication made him feel drowsy and less alert. I hated seeing him in pain. Eventually, I convinced him to keep a steady level of medication in his system and with the right combination of medication, he was able to enjoy most of his waking hours without feeling groggy and tired.

I started to wonder how much more his body could take. The cancer had spread to his lungs, brain, and bones. The best the medical community could offer was to manage the pain in the knee area and continue with chemotherapy as long as the disease was stable in the lungs and brain. There was nothing more they could do. The gravity of the situation continued to deepen each day. The worst that can happen was really yet to come. Soon he would no longer have any treatment.

Life is not the way it is supposed to be. It's the way it is. The way you cope with it is what makes the difference.

~ Virginia Satir, American author and psychotherapist

REFLECTION

There was a big disconnect between what I imagined it was like when someone was diagnosed with cancer, and the reality of when it happens to someone you love. When Callum was first diagnosed, I never imagined the barrage of medical issues to deal with when the cancer metastasized. Especially when so much happened in such a short time.

I definitely never thought that at forty-seven years old I would be told my husband was dying. We really had just started living. That was the number one lesson I learned. Life isn't fair. All too soon my husband would die. Frankly. That was the worst that could happen.

TIPS

1. Be Prepared. Go into every doctor appointment expecting to hear the worst news. If it happens, you are ready. If it doesn't, you feel better.
2. Know your reality. If your loved one has a terminal diagnosis, be real about it. You don't have to dwell on it. Experience every kind of joy and happiness possible. Make every moment count.
3. Suggested ways to cope/stress busters:
    a. Write in a journal
    b. See the social worker at the Cancer Centre/Hospital
    c. See a psychologist/counsellor/coach.
    d. Look for a caregiver support group in your area.
    e. Call a friend.
    f. Take a nap.
    g. Take a warm bath.
    h. Read an inspirational and uplifting story.

TIME FOR YOUR REFLECTION

1. What kind of unexpected crises have you had on your caregiver journey?
2. What has helped you get through them?
3. What did you try that didn't help?

Chapter Five

The Centre Of The Universe

Dream as if you'll live forever. Live as though you'll die tomorrow.

~ James Dean, American actor

When Callum was diagnosed with terminal cancer, my outlook on life immediately changed. With his mortality staring us square in the face, I saw our life together being cut short. There was no time to play around with being petty, nor time to sweat the small stuff. It was time to hurry up and get things done. When I stepped into being his caregiver on a grander scale, my perspective shifted again. Priorities changed, the important things rose to the top, and I really didn't care what was on television. I considered the time Callum and I had left together as our retirement—our future I used to think was years away. Our life was now on fast-forward, and I was going to make damn sure we enjoyed it. When his life expectancy was shortened to a year or less, the real pressure was on. Packing twenty or thirty years of living into three years was a challenge. Cramming it into less than a year created a vortex of frenzy and soon my plans to see Callum achieve his dreams became the centre of our universe—the centre of my universe.

Time was precious and not to be wasted. The expectations of our family changed dramatically over three years. He had his bucket list, and I had my list of things I wanted to enjoy doing with him. As we checked off what was accomplished, the trip to Scotland, buying the Porsche, seeing AC/DC, we added more to the list. I truly believed we needed to keep setting goals a few months ahead. It helped to bring him hope and more determination to live.

During the first few months after Callum was first diagnosed with cancer, the main mission was to get through treatment and surgery. When there was no further evidence of disease, our life returned to normal and it was easier to set goals and attend to the bucket list.

The universe started to shift in January 2008. The momentum was already building in our personal lives. Vanessa's wedding, new jobs, and finding a house created a sense of urgency that escalated from that time on. These were major life changes in their own right. Thrown into the mix were new medical issues faced by Callum. There was no down time.

That summer I was still coming to terms with the inevitable death of my husband. The increasing deterioration of his health and unpredictable crises created anxiety and urgency. The stress meter went up a few notches. My passion was to help him live, really live, as great a life he could in the time he had left. Aside from a few bucket list items, his priority was spending time with family and friends. There was no shortage of those who wanted to spend time with him. The challenge became finding a balance. With all those visitors, time for us as a couple—and the quiet time Callum and I needed for rest and recovery during and after treatment cycles—were hard to come by. Yet there were times when other people were necessary players in achieving many of our goals.

When it was time, these people stepped up to the plate. They were all willing to be part of what Callum wanted to do, see, or experience. Some had serious thoughts of self-sacrifice in order to make his dreams come true.

Shortly before Callum started chemotherapy in May 2008, Vanessa and Stuart were visiting us in Saskatoon. Callum got Vanessa and I complementary tickets for Phantom of the Opera from his employer, the *StarPhoenix* newspaper. The newspaper had box seats, and when we entered the box, a lovely tray of vegetables with dip, fruit, cheese, and crackers greeted us, along with a bottle of white wine for Vanessa, a bottle of red for me. We giggled with the luxury and elegance of the moment. My favourite part was the cup holders in our seats. I felt like royalty being able to sip on wine while enjoying the performance.

Vanessa and I talked about how we were feeling about the news that Callum had terminal cancer. The conversation led to the sensitive topic of grandchildren. Vanessa and Stuart were married only four months by this time. It was a big thing for me to ask if they would consider having a child––Callum's grandchild. To my surprise, Vanessa had been thinking the same thing.

"Stuart and I have talked about whether or not we should have a baby," she explained. "It's a big decision."

"It is," I agreed. "I feel really selfish asking you to do this. I know your dad would absolutely do anything to be a granddad. The catch is, after he dies, you and Stuart will still be parents. It is a huge commitment."

"I know. It's a lot to ask of Stuart. He's only twenty-four. It is a big difference that he's two years younger than me. I'm not sure he's ready to be a dad," she continued.

"I can only tell you how much it would mean to your dad if he could be a granddad. I am full of mixed emotions and don't want you to feel like I am forcing anything on you," I added.

"I know. We are thinking about it. We haven't really planned to have a baby so soon. But I want my child to know their granddad. That is really important to me," she said emphatically.

That was how it was left. We agreed on the magnitude of the importance of a grandchild for Callum. Vanessa and I also knew that he wouldn't want her to get pregnant just so he could be a granddad. He would never have asked her to do that. I would. I did. It felt selfish. But this wasn't about me.

He had a deep desire to be a granddad and was convinced this wouldn't happen. He didn't know how much his love and commitment to family had been passed on to our daughter, Vanessa. But after that conversation, I let it slide. The rest of the year I was busy dealing with the many sudden medical crises, and my focus turned to providing emotional and physical support to Callum—and to doing some of the things I knew would make him happy.

The diagnosis of the brain tumours and shortened life expectancy ramped up the urgency to do as much as possible while Callum was still able. We were committed to spending time with family as much as possible.

Val and Ray, my sister and brother-in-law, bought a house in Ixtapa, Mexico, in 2008. By late October the renovations were finished, and they were ready to spend their first winter there. Believing Callum would not live another winter, we jumped at the chance to take a last minute trip to see them. One thing on his bucket list was to go deep-sea fishing and Ixtapa was the perfect destination.

When we arrived in Ixtapa, Callum was fatigued and at times nauseous from the effects of radiation and chemotherapy. We carefully planned the week so that he could rest as much as possible and still enjoy a vacation. Deep-sea fishing was the priority and Callum was pumped up with anticipation. It warmed my heart to see him excited and lively about something. There hadn't been much for us to cheer about lately.

Ray and Callum decided Wednesday would be the day to go fishing. They headed to the beach and found a fellow Canadian who offered deep-sea fishing trips. It was off-season; they got a wicked deal and set out on the ocean. It wasn't long before they caught two small tuna and a seven-foot sailfish. Up next, the marlin. It was quite a catch! On the hook was a 180 pound, nine-foot long blue marlin! Callum was exhilarated.

The "boys" came into the house, huge grins plastered on their faces.

"I've caught my big fish, " Callum exclaimed. "It was amazing. Those guys knew exactly where to go to get it."

I was thrilled to see Callum so happy. It had been a really tough month. He had his driver's license revoked because of the brain tumours and would soon be on long-term disability. It had been a long time since I'd seen him smile. The joy he got from catching the marlin was worth every penny the trip cost.

It was an adventure Callum wouldn't forget. I was grateful that Ray made it happen, even though he didn't like fishing. He did it for Callum.

We had a fabulous week floating in their pool, going to the beach, and having authentic Mexican meals. It was a nice break for me. Ray kept Callum out of my hair, and I enjoyed some well-deserved relaxation time hanging out with my sister in the pool. When it came time to say good-bye, we were all hit by a sense of reality. You could have cut the tension around us with a knife. Tears filled everyone's eyes as we stood together at the airport. Each one of us was thinking it, This would likely be the last time Val and Ray would see Callum alive. No one spoke it. The thought kept poking and prodding at my brain. The urge to keep things positive overcame the thought. I couldn't comprehend that the next time I would see Val and Ray I might be alone, a widow. There was so much gratitude for having family who wanted to help Callum tick off his bucket list. There was fear, sadness, and despair knowing it might be the last time we'd all be together. We put on our fake smiles, pretended this was an ordinary good-bye, and exchanged hugs and kisses.

The frenzy was starting to build.

The longer Callum lived, the greater the urgency I had to help him accomplish what he wanted. With only months to live, I pushed and pushed to have something to look forward to. I had no idea that I was in for a marathon. The first few months after treatment for the brain metastases were intense. I remembered hearing that the cancer journey was a roller coaster, full of ups and downs. There was something missing in that analogy. The journey may be a roller coaster with high times and low times. The stress doesn't end. It doesn't slow down. If things are going sideways health wise, there is stress and worry that the end is near. If things are going well, there is stress wondering when it will suddenly end. The stress steadily, day by day, minute by minute increased. I don't remember noticing it happening at the time.

Looking back, I realize what happened is that each time I reached a new level of stress, I maintained it until it became normal. Then the next crisis would happen, the stress increased, and that level became normal. Eventually my normal state was to be extremely stressed and on high alert for anything, good or bad.

Each time the stress plateaued, I had a glimpse of what might be described as normal days. Get up, have breakfast, go to work, come home, get ready for the next day, go to bed. I desperately needed these days for recuperation from the constant worry and stress. I could rejuvenate and regain strength, maybe even lessen the stress. I could always hope this would happen.

As a rule, we stayed away from having visitors on the "chemo weekend," which was every second weekend. I had enough on my plate those weekends keeping up with meals, groceries, laundry, and getting Callum whatever would make him most comfortable. He spent a lot of time resting and sleeping. These were moments I took advantage of that and would sometimes catch a nap of my own. It was necessary because the good weekends were usually spent in Medicine Hat or with us hosting company in Saskatoon.

Every month the urgency of visits increased. I wanted to make each minute really count and now had only, at best, half the days in the month to make it happen. This urgency became contagious. When someone would call about coming to visit, I literally had to book them in. Everyone learned to give me lots of advance notice.

The cycle of frenzy bounced back and forth between living each moment as it were the last and planning things far enough in the future to have something to look forward to achieving. I'd look three to six months ahead and offer Callum some options for events, trips, or visits coming up.

As Callum became sicker and we started to expect that the cancer spread, I had to say, "Let's look at this after the next doctor's appointment." Neither of us wanted to be disappointed if we couldn't follow through on what we hoped to do.

I became a gatherer of special people and special moments. My life was on the fast track trying to fit in as much as possible in three-month increments. I kept my eyes and ears open for anything I knew Callum would enjoy. When I noticed upcoming events, trips to take, or people to visit, I would check the date, compare it to the current chemo schedule, and make arrangements for as many events as possible. We planned family get-togethers for holidays and birthdays. There was not likely going to be another chance to spend these special times together.

The race was on to get through the list before Callum was no longer able to do what he wanted. This whirlwind of activity continued for nearly three years. Once one thing was done, another was being planned. Sometimes that happened simultaneously.

Added to the frenzy of planning the bucket list was working around the schedule of chemotherapy. Sometimes things were important enough for the chemo schedule to be adjusted around what we were doing. I did my best to plan around chemotherapy and other medical tests. Some things, like the family vacation to Scotland and the AC/DC concert in Las Vegas, were priorities over chemotherapy, even though it was Callum's lifeline. The sad reality was that a shift of a week or two in treatment would not have an effect on the eventual outcome. Creating the life of his dreams took precedence.

I had to be relentless in all this planning. That was the only future I wanted to think about. Once there was no more planning for the two of us, I would be planning for only me. That was a scary thought. Those thoughts invoked feelings too overwhelming for me to deal with. I just couldn't go there. I didn't want to imagine what life was going to be like living alone.

The days and months went by and more and more I brought others into my frenzy. Callum's brother and his wife came to visit at least once every three months. Jamie travelled from Calgary to either Saskatoon or Medicine Hat to visit us once or twice a month. We travelled to Medicine Hat to visit Vanessa once or twice a month. Callum's parents came to visit two or three times a year. My sisters and their husbands visited twice a year. We had many friends visit. We made every reasonable attempt to attend any weddings, anniversaries, and birthday celebrations. Many holidays and birthdays were planned around Callum's health and treatment schedule. His life would soon end. There was not a minute to waste.

Life is an opportunity, benefit from it. Life is beauty, admire it. Life is bliss, taste it. Life is a dream, realize it. Life is a challenge, meet it. Life is a game, play it. Life is a promise, fulfill it. Life is sorrow, overcome it. Life is a song, sing it. Life is an adventure, dare it. Life is luck, make it. Life is too precious, do not destroy it.
Life is life, fight for it!

~ Mother Teresa

REFLECTION

Each time we were with family, the sense of urgency was heightened with the underlying thought that this could be the last family time with Callum. By the time he passed away, I had lost my ability to look any further than the next day or week. I didn't have a lot of patience to begin with and the years of having to do everything "now,"–because I didn't know if there would be another chance–only compounded my impatience.

I was doing the best I could at the time, keeping Callum as the centre of my universe.

TIPS

1. Find time every day for yourself, ten minutes at a minimum, twenty minutes is better. It will re-energize you.
2. Talk with your loved one about the balance they want among visiting, doing fun things, spending time with family, and having time to recover from treatment.
3. Let people know when important things are happening so they can decide if they want to take part.

TIME FOR YOUR REFLECTION

1. What are some ways you make sure to pace yourself when things start spinning out of control?
2. Do you think about things as, "This could be the last time _____________." Does it change your enjoyment of special moments when you worry it could be a "last time?"
3. What differences have you noticed in interactions with family and friends during this time?

Chapter Six

Life Is Meant To Be Lived

Maybe all one can do is hope to end up with the right regrets.

~ Arthur Miller, American playwright and essayist.

There was never a shortage of challenges living with Callum while he fought terminal cancer. I never knew what surprise was waiting just around the corner. There was no telling when things would get worse. There was no predicting when it all would be over. That was why it was so important; we captured every opportunity and lived every possible moment in peace, hope, and joy. Life is meant to be lived—not fretted away.

Each step Callum and I took in the cancer journey brought us closer together as a couple and as best friends. We had grown closer and our relationship became stronger after the children left home and we moved to Alberta. The cancer diagnosis intensified our relationship and took it to a whole new level. There was nothing worth fighting over anymore. I learned to be grateful for every moment we had together. I was not going to let him die without enjoying life. Thank goodness he had the same outlook. I was determined to create as much joy and happiness for him as possible.

One of the life changing and life affirming moments for me was when I was introduced to The Passion Test®. What really spoke to me was Janet Bray-Attwood's story about changing plans to live out her dream passion of going to India so that she could stay in the United States and care for her terminally ill stepmother. In her story, she explained that her family was also her passion, and she could put the India trip on hold in order to care for her stepmother. This was exactly the message I needed to hear. I wasn't losing myself. I didn't have to fight the intense focus of caregiving so I could be who I really was. I found permission for me to make caregiving for Callum my passion. This was a pivotal moment for me, and I never looked back. We were going to have the best life we could possibly have. I chose to go into debt in order to do as much as possible in the time we had left together. I justified this decision because I could pay off the debt with insurance money after he passed away. He was never going to have a normal retirement. I was not going to have the enjoyment of sharing retirement years with him. This was our only shot at enjoying some of those retirement moments together.

By the summer of 2006, Callum had healed from surgery. We slowly got back into a normal routine, especially with weekend golf. Plans were underway for our Scottish holiday a few months away. His Nana turned ninety that summer, and it was very important to him to visit her so that he could show her in person that he was OK. He didn't want her to worry. He didn't say it out loud, but I think it was really important to him that he took time to be with family and emotionally reconnect with his homeland. I wasn't going to stand in his way and quite enjoyed having something fun to look forward to and plan.

In the midst of the rounds of golf and holiday planning, we received a phone call from Stuart, our daughter's boyfriend.

"Hi, Mrs. Scott, May I speak with Mr. Scott, please?" he asked.

I replied, "Sure. Here he is." I handed the phone to Callum.

Intently, I watched his face for clues as he listened to Stuart. His eyes started to fill with tears and his chin started to quiver. I was pretty sure I knew what was happening and burst with excitement.

"I would be proud and excited for you to ask Vanessa to marry you. Thank you for asking my permission. We would be very happy to have you join our family," Callum managed to say, his voice breaking up as he spoke.

Our baby girl was going to get engaged in a few days! We were so excited. Stuart was a gentleman, and we knew he loved her very much. Callum never showed a lot of range in his emotions. When I saw his quivering chin and tears trickling down his face, I knew something had deeply touched his heart. This was one of those moments that gave us joy, hope, and another important reason for him to kick cancer's ass. Regardless of what was going to happen in the future, he was determined to be in the Dominican Republic to see our daughter get married.

In the months leading up to the wedding, I was relieved to hear at each doctor appointment that the cancer was under control. The slow growth of spots in one lung had caused us some concern, but there wasn't any reason to worry until they grew big enough to biopsy. We set that concern aside and focused on wedding plans and moving to Saskatoon. I loved looking forward to the wedding. When the darkness of worry about the lung spots crept in, the excitement of wedding plans helped shift me back to joy and hope.

We left Saskatoon on a frosty day in January 2008 and arrived in the Dominican Republic to bright sunshine and sprinkles of rain. I was thrilled that we woke up to a picture perfect day for the wedding. I'm sure Callum and his dad, Walter, were thinking it could have been a wee bit cooler for them as they were wearing wool kilts. It was worth it. Both of them beamed with pride, dressed in their Scott tartan kilts as they walked Vanessa to the gazebo where Stuart waited for his bride-to-be. Callum, with the quiver in his chin, lovingly, with pride and joy, wrapped his arms around Vanessa, gave her a huge hug and put her hand in Stuart's hand. My heart skipped a beat as I thought of how lucky we were that he was there to see Vanessa married. Under normal circumstances this would have been a very emotional moment. Coming face to face with Callum's mortality deepened the appreciation of being able to make the trip and amplified the joy of the moment. Each of us would treasure this very special time.

The marriage celebration continued a few months later when the reception was held in Medicine Hat. This was great practice for learning to find joy and hope when things looked bleak. The reception was sandwiched between learning Callum had terminal cancer and the start of chemotherapy. This could have been enough to drive one crazy. My emotions were all over the place. First, I was excited about planning decorations and food; then I was suddenly overcome with sadness thinking about his all too short life expectancy. I carried on. I was determined to keep this a happy time in our lives. There was no reason to dwell on what we couldn't control. The cancer would do whatever it would do. It was time to celebrate life!

Though the reception was a casual affair, Vanessa and Stuart planned a few formal moments. The bride and groom dance was special. Vanessa and Stuart looked like they just stepped off the plane from the Dominican Republic. I looked at Vanessa, who was absolutely gorgeous in her wedding dress, and Stuart, who was equally handsome in his beige pants and white shirt. The love they share was evident as they looked deep into each other's eyes while they danced. The next song came on and Vanessa lovingly took Callum to the middle of the dance floor. It was time for the traditional father-daughter dance. There were few dry eyes in the room. He smiled from ear to ear as he effortlessly guided Vanessa around the dance floor. They willingly and graciously paused for photos. That was a lifetime moment to be captured and remembered. The bubble of the fairy tale moment protected me from the harsh reality of my future. There would be plenty of time later to deal with that. What mattered most was that we were there, Callum and I, partying with our family and friends, celebrating the marriage of our daughter.

Later that fall he underwent the whole brain radiation treatment. I began to feel anxious about all the things he would miss after he passed away. Christmas time was approaching and he was getting weaker and weaker. The future was discouraging. I had to be honest with myself and knew it was time to prepare for his last Christmas. I didn't want a sad Christmas. I wanted a joyous Christmas. I did my best to keep it upbeat and consciously created a happy time.

As Christmas drew near we were surrounded by the presence and love of our family–Vanessa and Stuart, Jamie, Callum's parents, his brother Alan and wife Dorothy. Callum was an excellent host and graced us with a succulent rib eye roast for dinner on Christmas Eve. Bread and butter pudding topped off the meal, and we enjoyed this precious time together. I loved Christmas. I felt saddened that this would likely be the last Christmas we would share with him.

Christmas morning we woke up, grabbed some coffee, and eyed the presents around the tree. We were all spoiled! Our family tradition was for the kids to open their stockings and then hand out presents to the rest of us. We bought ourselves a video camera for Christmas so I watched the excitement of gift opening from behind the lens.

A few minutes into the throes of unwrapping, Stuart gently poked Vanessa, who looked up at Callum. I had a sense that something special was about to happen. I quickly moved the camera to him. He was holding a gift. All eyes were on Callum as he unwrapped it. He took a few seconds to carefully look it over. It was a photo frame that said: "Grandkisses ... Grandcuddles …Grandchild" and in the photo space in the frame was a picture of a stork carrying a baby, and the words: "I will arrive on June 27, 2009."

Callum looked at the piece of paper in the frame, lifted his head, and peered across the room at Vanessa.

"Are you pregnant?" he asked.

With tears in her eyes, she said, "Yes, I am."

Immediately Callum burst into tears. Vanessa crossed the room and gave him a hug. He took off his glasses to wipe his eyes, and his whole body shook with each sob. I stood there, behind the video camera, trying to catch up on what just happened. My baby was going to have a baby! I was going to be a grandma. Callum was going to be a granddad. He wanted so much to be a granddad. Now he had a chance. The tough part would be living long enough to see his grandchild.

The next few months flew by, and Callum started to recover from the effects of radiation. I was convinced that this grandchild-to-be gave him renewed determination to live. It gave the rest of us hope that we would have him in our lives a little longer.

On July 7, 2009, 4:17 a.m., Cade Scott Bonneville was born. Callum and I were able to see him when he was only minutes old. I was bursting with excitement and joy. For months, deep down I was afraid to believe that he would be here for Cade's birth. I kept pushing back the fear and focused on hope. I couldn't bear the thought of this joyful moment without him. I was grateful it didn't happen that way. Stuart gently placed Cade into Callum's arms. His smile lit up the room. A few tears trickled down his face and he lovingly examined every inch of Cade's face. There wasn't much time to hold Cade right then. It had been a tricky delivery and Cade needed to get into the NICU (neo-natal intensive care unit) to warm up. We were lucky to share another of life's precious moments.

That gift, our darling grandson, not only renewed Callum's fight for life, but gave us the gift of two more "last Christmases." He lived to celebrate Cade's second birthday. It was our miracle that he should live two years longer than anyone thought was possible.

Living in a world where every life milestone could be the last, I made sure we celebrated and enjoyed every opportunity we could. In 2011, Callum and I both turned fifty. Most people at this time of their life would be starting to seriously think about retirement and how they would enjoy those years together. My hope and dream was that he lived three months past his birthday to celebrate my fiftieth birthday.

Callum's birthday was January 14th and plans were underway to surprise him with a birthday tea with his friends, followed by a supper with family and close friends. This was difficult when we spent pretty much every single minute together. Thankfully, I was able to use some time at work in my office and could make some of the arrangements without him finding out. A very important thing I wanted that day was to have professional family photos done. I thought he still looked pretty good, and it was a great reason to be dressed up. The family photo shoot became the excuse to get him to the hall for his birthday tea.

It had been only ten days since Callum made the serious decision to go ahead with surgery to remove the brain tumour. Surgery was only two weeks after the party. Life was not settled at all and there was an air of worry that surrounded us. It did not overtake us. I was determined to celebrate life.

The family pitched in to run errands and help decorate the hall for the birthday tea. The family photo shoot took place just before the tea. We started with the whole family, all six of us: Callum, Jamie, Vanessa, Stuart, Cade, and me. Cade was eighteen months old, and sometimes it was a challenge to keep him still and smiling. The family photo from two years earlier didn't have Cade in it, and I wanted one before Callum became sicker. The dress code for the day was black and red which nicely complemented Callum's kilt. I sat there with pride in my heart, knowing our wonderful family would have a great keepsake. There were moments I had to work hard to not cry. Cade gave us some comic relief, and it kept Callum busy while people were arriving. Butterflies bounced all around in my stomach, and I hoped we would keep the surprise as long as possible.

The plan worked great. That was up until some early birds arrived, and he happened to meet them at the entrance. He thought it was a big coincidence that Linda and Ray were in the same place—until they said "Happy Birthday." He quickly figured it out. I took him over to the hall. He walked in the door and saw the guest book table. He took a few more steps into the room and noticed all the balloon centrepieces. Bright, colourful balloons. It was a birthday party! He smiled from ear to ear.

"This is for me?" he asked with excitement.

"Yes, it is," I lovingly answered.

"Really?" he asked again. "I thought this was for someone else. I figured out we were having a family supper, but I never thought anything else was happening. I am very surprised," he said with a giggle.

"You never expected this?" I said with astonishment. "I thought you might have known about all of it by now."

"No. I caught on that my family was coming and we'd have supper," he said. Then he took in the whole room, moving his gaze to take it all in. "That's set up for a lot of people. You did all this—for me?"

My eyes looked straight into his as I said, "Yes, happy birthday, sweetheart."

We gave each other a warm embrace and shared tears of joy, love, and hope.

My mission was accomplished. I wanted to give him a better party than he could imagine. Guests came from four provinces covering many miles. Callum was blown away by the more than seventy-five people at the tea. He expressed his humility and gratitude in his thank you speech:

All I really wanted to say was, the important people in our lives, and really everything didn't start to pick up until we moved west here. And that's when things started to happen. And I think that's a testament to the people in this room today. 'Cause most of them are from this area. All I really want to say is thanks for coming this afternoon. I know there's been a lot of kidding and a lot of joking, and a lot of that stuff. And I really appreciate that. We're looking forward to moving back down here, being closer to the kids, and closer to everything that's important to us. We're really looking forward to that. People have come from a long ways away. This is a surprise. I mean the fact that you folks and Lorna did all the hard work to make this come together, it's just amazing. To have this many people it's amazing, It just blows me away (he chokes) you have to choke on it. I'm a very humble person. Some of the quotes were true and we've got people from all over the place, and I think that's just amazing. All of you guys deserve a pat on the back for being able to make it because I sure as heck wouldn't have come here in this weather!

Jamie and Vanessa entertained us with the top ten things they learned as Callum's children. Number one was:

"Life isn't fair. But it's to be lived to the fullest. The best gift we can all give my dad today, is to do that, and live our own lives to the fullest."

There was no doubt our time with Callum was limited. He was in extreme pain from the bone metastases and it was frightening knowing the brain tumour was growing again. I could have thrown in the towel and babied him. We could have sat around together, thinking about all the "what if's." Not us. Life is meant to be lived to the fullest. There were many things to celebrate and enjoy.

On my birthday, Jamie drove from Calgary to Medicine Hat to be with us. I was grateful that Vanessa, Stuart, Cade, and Jamie joined Callum and me for my birthday dinner. That was the first time I had seen a twenty-month old child enjoy shrimp! Cade already learned to enjoy the finer things in life. I had so much joy with him. Yet behind the joy I was feeling there was a sense of dread. I wasn't looking forward to the next day. Callum had an appointment with Dr. Haider, and we knew there was a good possibility the cancer had started to grow and his treatment would end. Each one of us sat there, happy faces glued on, pretending that we were a regular family having a regular birthday celebration.

The next day we found out Callum was no longer responding to chemotherapy and all treatment would be halted.

My fiftieth birthday gave me an opportunity to reflect on what I had learned over fifty years. I shared this with others through my blog, "Walking the Journey Together . . . Alone" (www.calupdate.blogspot.com):

On April 4th, I move from one decade to the next. The big "50!" I can remember when only old people turned 50—how did we all become so young at 50? It has been quite the fun times over the past 50 years. There have certainly been some very sad times, some troublesome times, and some anxious moments. But we have always tried to keep some fun in there somewhere. I think I am almost old enough now to know that I really "don't know it all," and likely never will.

I have learned the power of love and hope. And I have learned that the power of love comes in all ways—and sometimes most of all through the pain of having to renew it again. But love will win in the end.

I have learned (and really try hard to practice!) to not judge.

I have learned that giving people a hand up can sometimes help more than a hand out. That most people want to be successful, but sometimes just lack the tools and knowledge to get there. And sometimes people are extremely happy with their lives, even though we might not be if it were us—and that is OK.

I have learned that most parents want to be good parents—they just don't know how. It is pure joy to see a mom try something new with her baby and see it work. Smiles on both mom and babe light up a room!

Everyone has strengths—look for them, nurture them, grow them—in you, and in others.

I have learned the importance of being honest, doing a good job, and working hard. Compassion and understanding go a long way.

I have learned that it is important to find out who you are, what are your values, and then matching these to all your activities—work, volunteer, hobbies, friendships.

When you have lost your strength—don't be afraid to ask for help, from family, friends, medical professionals, and from whatever you use for faith.

I am still learning the power of patience—and that learning is a life long process. Enjoy it!

I have learned that what you have now won't last forever. Not the couch, the computer, the flowers, your clothes. And that special people in your life leave this world far too early.

I have learned how quickly things can change in a minute. I have learned the positive side of being stubborn, determined, persistent, and perhaps, even obstinate.

I have learned that no matter what are your troubles, everyone has troubles. They are not to be measured against each other—the biggest challenge in someone's life is still their biggest challenge. Honour it.

I have learned that being kind, even to the nastiest person, is still better than being nasty. I don't believe anyone really feels better when they act nasty.

I have learned that family can move about and be miles away from each other, but are always there when you need them.

I have learned that if you keep your eyes and ears open you will find opportunities you never thought existed. Sometimes you need to close your mouth so you can see and hear them.

I have learned that yes, you can love someone even more tomorrow. And that you can pack in 50-60 years of loving in thirty.

My 50th birthday wish is that you take time to tell those special people you love them and miss them. Pick up the phone or email a friend or family who you have not spoken with for a while. Take time for yourself. Cherish and be grateful for all the wonderful, beautiful things you have in your life.

For ten years I had wanted to have my fiftieth birthday supper at Tavern on the Green in Central Park, New York City. By 2011, Tavern on the Green had closed. I hoped against all hope that we would make it to the Big Apple and find a better place for my birthday dinner. I had given up a lot over the last few years and was going to give up even more when Callum died. I thought it was only fair, that somehow, I'd get a Make-A-Wish. Callum bounced between telling me to take a look at making plans, and weeping because he knew there was no way he was well enough for that trip. I knew he wanted to keep the hope alive for me. It just wasn't in the cards.

My family joined me in planning my birthday party two weeks later. It was a wonderful day. I entered the hall to Frank Sinatra belting out "New York, New York." Somehow, they found a bakery who made fresh New York Style pretzels. To top it off, I sipped on Cosmopolitan cocktails all night. One of my favourite shows was *Sex and the City*, and Carrie always drank Cosmopolitans. It was my dream that I'd celebrate my fiftieth birthday in New York City, and after dinner, I would go to a jazz club and drink Cosmopolitans. I was blessed to have so many people I loved work so hard to give me a piece of my dream.

Callum had others look after him that night. I laughed, drank, and danced the night away. I couldn't remember the last time I had that much fun. My ten-year dream of a New York City celebration was dead. With the care and compassion of friends and family, I had a birthday party I wouldn't forget. I'm glad we took the time to celebrate. And as I looked at my family, I knew that Callum, and I had done well, particularly with our kids.

Callum was proud of his children. That really was an understatement. I don't know if Jamie and Vanessa ever understood the depths of his love, pride, and joy for them. They are marvellous adults and gave him many reasons to be a proud dad.

Vanessa studied hard the last few years and passed her final exam to become a Chartered Accountant. It wasn't an easy road for her, which made the accomplishment that much sweeter. The icing on the cake was that Callum and I would be at the ceremony and ball to see her presented with her certificate. He wouldn't have it any other way. He fought nausea, headaches, and pain just to be there. I couldn't tell who was more thrilled that he was there, Vanessa or him. This was a treasured time in a relationship between father and daughter. Callum was proud of Vanessa's determination, perseverance, and success. Vanessa was proud of herself for the same things, and was lovingly grateful her dad was in the audience to see this happen. I, too, was proud and soaked in all the love and gratitude. I was overwhelmed with joy and love when I stood back and watched them share this wonderful moment. We were all proud of her. Nothing compares to that special father-daughter bond.

Jamie and Callum shared a love for golf. He was a good golfer and Jamie was even better. Jamie enjoyed a pretty good amateur golf career and Callum was there to support him as much as possible. There are four "major" amateur tournaments in Medicine Hat and by 2010 Jamie had won all of them but one. The Victoria Day Classic had been just out of reach for him. Jamie set a goal to win the 2011 Victoria Day tournament. He practiced and practiced all winter long. Callum and I knew nothing about his goal or his plans to dedicate this tournament win to his dad.

It was a rainy afternoon on the third and final round of the 2011 Victoria Day Classic. Jamie was in the hunt for the win. The rain fell harder and harder and play was suspended. Everyone went scurrying into the clubhouse to wait for it to clear up. It was quite a downpour and the course quickly filled up with puddles. The tournament committee decided to cancel the rest of the round. They awarded prizes based on the scores from the first two rounds to everyone, except the champion. Jamie was tied for first place with Scott Desmarais. A champion had to be crowned. They went back out to hole number ten for a playoff. After a wayward drive, Jamie hit a spectacular second shot, made his putt for birdie, and won the tournament. During media interviews, and in his acceptance speech, he publicly acknowledged that he played to win this for his dad. Nothing compares to that special father-son bond.

Family moments and celebrations were high up on the list of memories I wanted to create. Fun times. Loving times. Times that brought us hope. Times of great joy. The top three things in Callum's life were family, golf, and music. That was why live music concerts were on his list of things to do. Saskatoon was a regular stop for some of Callum's favourite bands. I love live music and got even more pleasure sharing this with him. We enjoyed watching John Mellencamp, Neil Young, Leonard Cohen, and ZZ Top, to name a few. Two bands high on Callum's list to see were AC/DC and U2. It took me a bit of maneuvering to make it happen.

Not so lucky for AC/DC, and lucky for us, they had to reschedule their 2009 fall tour to the spring of 2010. I found some tickets, booked our flights, and we were off to Las Vegas. Callum was a trooper on the trip, even when he hobbled around with a sore leg. That didn't stop him from being thrilled to see AC/DC live in concert. I loved making his wishes come true.

Nearly two months after being told the cancer was no longer controlled, I dragged him to Edmonton to see U2. Persistence helped. U2 also had to cancel their tour the year before so it was a wait to see them. Callum wasn't sure whether he should be making this trip. He was using a wheelchair anytime we were out. He was worried about getting to and from the stadium. I had it all under control. A hotel room, a cab, a wheelchair, and we were set! It actually made some things easier, since there was special treatment at concerts for anyone in a wheelchair. No lines to wait in. We got to go past everyone and go right to our seats. The set was incredible and the music undeniably brilliant. The only hiccup we encountered was trying to get a cab after the concert. Jamie and I pushed Callum up and down the streets near Commonwealth Stadium for nearly two hours before we found a cab. We didn't get back to the hotel until 2:00 a.m. We ordered some pizza and went straight to bed. Not bad for a guy who passed away six weeks later.

I didn't leave anything to chance. I found out what Callum wanted to do. I asked him directly. When he didn't believe it could happen, I found a way to help him believe it was possible. Once that was done, the resources for us to make it happen showed up.

One of Callum's dreams, for as long as many people remembered, was to drive a Porsche. Jamie had fond memories of him talking about it. In grade two, Vanessa drew pictures about a Porsche. Callum thought a Porsche was out of the question, knowing that he was dying. I was willing to make that dream come true. We had the good fortune of having a big income tax refund after moving to Saskatoon. This, I told him, could pay for a used Porsche. He started looking for one and in May 2009 he picked up his Black 2000 Porsche Boxster. Every minute he spent in that car was filled with joy and exhilaration.

We had a wild ride for those few years. And enjoyed every minute we lived it.

Life was meant to be lived, and curiosity must be kept alive.
One must never, for whatever reason, turn his back on life.

~ Eleanor Roosevelt, longest serving First Lady of U.S.A.

REFLECTION

It took courage, planning, and yes, some sacrifice, to do these things for Callum. I could have hoarded the insurance money. He might have had more rest that way! He would have not had the joy though. I would not have had the joy. We would not have had the joy. I am grateful that we grabbed every opportunity to fill the moments with joy and hope. Callum taught me to live life to the fullest.

TIPS

1. Make a list of the favourite things your loved one enjoys and would like to do. Include all dreams and wishes, even if they seem not possible. Prioritize the list and make plans to start doing them.

2. If finances are an issue in order to carry out some final wishes, there are options. Let others know of the wishes. There are people who are willing to help. Some other ideas are:
    a. Friends/family can hold a fundraiser for you.
    b. Look for donation funding websites, such as www.gofundme.com
    c. Research agencies and organizations who grant wishes for dying people.
    d. Always plan for something in the future. Plan for one, two, and three months ahead. Find one or two things six to twelve months in the future to look forward to.
    e. Churches or other faith based institutions
    f. Service organizations
3. If you had one last chance to do something with your loved one, what would it be? What would be the next step you could take in doing it?

TIME FOR YOUR REFLECTION

1. Contemplate your values: What does your loved one value most? What do you value most? What are the values you share? What are the differences? What will it take for you to honour the values your loved one has that are different than yours?
2. What are the dreams you and your loved one share? What do you need to do to make them happen?
3. What are some of life's milestones coming up that can be turned into celebrations? Major birthdays? Anniversaries? Holidays?
    a. Who can help you make these events memorable? Consider any kind of help. It could be financial help or practical help. Do you need someone to travel with you? Do you need more income? What do you need to have happen so that you can make some dreams come true?

Chapter Seven

All Aboard

Help one another; there's no time like the present and no present like the time.

~ James Durst, poet, songwriter

The first months after Callum's diagnosis were challenging. We had new jobs, moved to a new city, and were building a new home. There was little time for the cancer dish served to him. That had to change. My schedule was suddenly turned upside down and I had to find a way to fit it in. New information and appointments were flying in all directions. We had to get clear on who was going to do what and when. Callum moved into the patient role, and I took on more of the regular responsibilities. I thought I could do it alone. I tried to do it alone. I couldn't.

The biggest lesson here was not only to ask for help, but be open to receive it. It began with being open with anyone and everyone who was involved in our lives.

One essential and challenging task was to stay on top of the building of our new house. Everything happened so fast in the last weeks of building that I was worried I would miss something, especially when we were in Calgary for Callum's treatment. That was my first step forward in asking. Communication with the builder was vital. I shared with them enough of what was happening so they understood why we didn't communicate daily and only caught up on the house progress on weekends. That wasn't a hard thing to ask for and I was thankful we found a way to make things work.

Between email for non-urgent things and phone calls when immediate answers were needed, we found the best solution for each of us.

As moving day approached, I was overwhelmed by the thought of moving everything from our apartment and storage unit into our house. When the day finally arrived, Callum's dad, Walter, stayed in Calgary with him, and I was left to be in charge of the move. My brother Gerald, sister Val, brother-in-law Ray, and my mother-in-law Mary, were helping me, 150 kilometres away in Red Deer. I was annoyed to admit I needed help. Callum and I should have been looking after this ourselves. That was how my world was supposed to be. I was frustrated that I had little energy and concentration to organize the move. That was the paradox. I hated asking for and needing help, and I was in a situation where I didn't even know where to begin to ask. Thankfully, help arrived anyway.

The staff who worked for Callum offered to put together a moving crew. I wasn't fully open to accept it. I was very uncomfortable. Somehow, I found the strength to step into humility and receive. I had no energy to do otherwise. To add fuel to the fire, there was a part of me that just didn't care. Without Callum to join me in the move, the excitement of moving into the house was gone. His absence just emphasized the possibility that I might one day live alone in the house.

At 6:00 p.m. Fred, the publisher of the newspaper and Callum's boss, picked up the keys to the apartment and the storage shed. In less than an hour, the first truck arrived. I looked outside and saw a line-up of seven trucks loaded with our belongings. Seventeen people helped that cold, wet night in November. One by one, the trucks backed into the garage, and the assembly line began. The trucks were unloaded piece by piece, box by box. The items were passed from one person to another, and into the house where another line of people waited to put everything in its place. It was an amazing evening. In two and a half hours, the crew packed up and delivered our entire household, had pizza and beer, and were gone. My family and I sat there, eyes wide open, jaws dropped, wondering what the hell just happened. Not one of my family, nor I, had any concept of the amazing things that the moving team would accomplish.

Even though I didn't like to accept help, that night I was grateful I gave in to it. I would have been in a puddle of tears had I tried to do all of that on my own. At first I felt like a charity case accepting this help. It didn't take long to feel a deep sense of relief. I found out how generous people could be, and when I allowed others to help, I felt better, and so did they.

People like to help those in need. It seems to be human nature. Ironically, it also seems to be human nature to want to do it all by ourselves. I had been independent as long as I could remember. I learned early on that I was responsible for making things happen if I wanted them to happen. I had a few disappointments when I let others help me. Asking for help does not come easily for most of us. That was true for Callum and me.

Callum and I were married young and had children early in our lives. We were underdogs in our own right and determined, perhaps even stubborn, wanting to show the world we could make it on our own. That determination carried us through the next thirty years, and by the time he was diagnosed with cancer, we hadn't really needed anyone's help anymore. The important lesson here was that our friends and family wanted to help. My job was to let them know how. I got to practice on his parents first.

Dependable, steady, and always willing to help was how I would describe Walter and Mary. They arrived shortly after he was diagnosed and were with us through the ups and downs of treatment and surgery. I was eager for their help. Neither Callum nor I seemed to be able to get through the day doing all the things we needed to do. By the time we got home from work, we looked at each other hoping the other had what it would take to make some kind of supper. We were ready to be looked after. Mary and Walter to the rescue. It didn't take long for my fantasy bubble to burst.

The first day Walter and Mary were there, I got home from work, looking forward to not having to think about supper. I opened the door and expected to smell something. There was no smell of food cooking. I looked at the counter, then the stove. There was no smell because nothing was cooking. "What did they do all day?" I asked myself.

"I was going to cook supper, but didn't know what you wanted," Mary explained.

I couldn't tell if I was more disappointed or angry. Food. Cook food. Why can't you think for yourself?

My outside voice said, "Oh, OK. I'll figure out something."

I had a hard enough time trying to figure out how to feed the two of us. How was I supposed to figure out how to feed four? I thought they were here to help. I now had two more people to look after. Parents are supposed to help their children. That was what I thought it was about. Momentarily, I forgot they were also deeply affected by Callum's cancer diagnosis. I took a step back emotionally and decided to look at the situation as if I was supervising staff at work. They needed clear expectations, the tools to do the job, and feedback on what would or wouldn't work. It took me a few days and I finally got to a point where I was brave and calm enough to have that conversation. I think it helped all of us to have this sorted out. Soon after we were looked after with emotional support and extra help with meals, laundry, groceries, and other household chores. I really appreciated the ease in the pressure of having to do it all myself and continuing to work. It still felt uncomfortable to need help. I was learning to let that go. It was a lot easier to let it go when I knew what to ask for and let others know what I needed.

With Callum's cancer diagnosis, nearly every moment was intense. Having Callum's parents with us helped us talk about some of the tough stuff and also gave us some diversion from that tough stuff. Over and over during the next six years, they were there for us. They provided a shoulder to cry on, practical help when needed, and hugs to ease the pain. The best gift I could give them was to let them help.

Over time I was more and more comfortable accepting help—especially when I knew Callum would not be cured, and would become more dependent on me as he got sicker.

Most of the time in the journey I knew in advance when help was needed. I could plan around surgery or our moves. Each time, I learned how to handle these situations even better. I believed I had it all under control. Suddenly one day I found out that I needed help—immediately.

Early on a cold January morning in 2010, Callum was not well. He had a headache, was nauseas, vomiting, and in a cold sweat so bad the bed was soaked. We were off to the emergency room where he started to spike a fever. I soon realized this was no ordinary stomach flu. His heart rate was high and his blood pressure was low. He was hooked up to machines to keep track of his vital signs. All of this commotion worried me. I was concerned that something was wrong with the brain tumour. It had been about a month since the last gamma knife treatment. Atavan was the only thing that stopped the shivering and kept him still enough for the CT scan of his brain. I was relieved that the results showed there was nothing to worry about. A few more tests were completed and an infection was found, but they were not sure what it was or how to treat it. Callum agreed to stay overnight until they could find out the source of the problem and make sure the broad spectrum antibiotic was working.

The next day, I found out that he had sepsis and would be in the hospital for another four or five days while they investigated and treated the infection. I remembered from my first aid training that sepsis was a very serious infection. That didn't matter. I had become complacent with the bumps in the road, and I underestimated the seriousness of this medical crisis. He had faced so many things and survived that I no longer winced when things seemed to go sideways.

He was quite tired and slept a lot during the day. I was used to a balancing act when it came to him and my job duties so I checked in on him in the morning and went to work for most of the day. Being at my office gave me a reprieve from the real world. I tried not to worry about him. I returned to the hospital mid afternoon and expected the next few days to be like this. Get up, go to the hospital, go to work, back to the hospital, go home, and go to bed. Pretty simple. And exhausting. As usual, I did what I had to do.

Thursday, January 29, 2010. I got to the hospital and enjoyed having breakfast with Callum. He was sitting in a chair and looked much better, and I could tell the antibiotics were working. It felt like a load had been taken off my shoulders, and I worried less about going to work during the day.

I returned to the hospital mid afternoon. Callum was sitting up in bed. He'd just finished a blood transfusion, and they were flushing the fluid build up out of him. He no longer could get to the bathroom fast enough and wet the bed. No big deal. It was just another one of those things that happened. I pulled an apple out of my backpack and started to eat it while they laid him down to change the bed and find clean pajamas. He started shivering and asked for another blanket and the oxygen. I covered him up and let the nurse know he wanted oxygen.

Next thing I knew I heard Callum yell out, "Ron, where are you Ron?"

I had no idea who Ron was, and thought he must have mixed up the name of the male nurse. I turned to look at him and saw his eyes rolling back in his head. I heard him struggle to breathe. I tied to stay calm, but inwardly I felt out of control. I yelled to the other nurse in the room, “He’s having trouble breathing, and his eyes are rolling back in his head!”

What happened right after that is a blur. I had just taken a bite of my apple, was standing at the foot of his bed, and then I watched as he tried to catch his breath. Without warning, I felt an arm across my shoulders and heard, “My name is Susan. I am the clinical nursing supervisor. You and Callum have been through a lot. Do you know if he wants to be intubated?”

“I have to decide that right now?” I asked with disbelief.

“Yes, you do,” Susan softly replied. “We need to know now, just

in case.”

My mind started jumping around. Intubation is life saving. If he needs that, it means his life is in danger. My mind jumped again. “My daughter is going to Mexico later today. Should I be telling her not to go?”

“I think that would be a good idea,” Susan advised.

My heart beat faster and faster, and I had trouble catching my breath. I went into the hallway and made my call to Vanessa. My hands shook as I pressed each number on the phone. I took a deep breath and was confident I would stay strong.

Vanessa answered the phone, “Hello.”

My voice cracked and I blurted, “Dad isn’t good and they say you shouldn’t go to Mexico.”

All I heard on the other end of the phone was crying. She heard the panic in my voice.

She got a grip on herself enough to say, “Should we be coming to Saskatoon?”

“Yes,” I managed to answer.

In less than fifteen minutes, I went from eating an apple and believing my husband was on his way to recovery to calling my daughter, asking her to cancel her belated honeymoon vacation because her dad had taken a turn for the worst. I could have used some help. I was not supposed to be alone when that happened. That was not how I thought it would be. I always thought I'd be surrounded by our families when Callum died. I knew this was not the time to be a hero and started to think about who to ask for help.

I felt like I was outside of myself, watching a movie. My thoughts took time to process.

I went back into his room and was alarmed to see him totally surrounded by people in white coats discussing what to do. One, two, three, four, five, six. Too many for me to count. All I could hear was Callum gasping for air. I was frozen in time and yet my mind raced. He has to be OK. He has fought too hard for it to end right now. I was not ready. We were not ready. I planned to write a book, and this was not how the story would end.

Someone came over to me and tried to talk to me while gently guiding me out of the room. I knew they needed space to work. I was terrified that if I left he would die when I was not there. I couldn't stay away for long. I had to go back in the room and talk to Sue.

"Should I be calling the family to come?" I asked, mustering up all the courage I could find.

"It is too early to tell for sure," Sue replied. "I would strongly encourage you to let them know what is happening."

I called Jamie. Thankfully, I caught him before he went to work that night. He assured me he would be on his way as soon as he could. He had a six-hour drive ahead of him.

The next closest family lived five hours away. They deserved notice. A wave of fear swept over me. Was this the end for Callum? I had no idea how to tell his family this news. I pulled out my cell phone, stared at it, and realized I had no daytime phone numbers for his family. His parents and sister-in-law were away at a meeting. I tried calling his brother Alan on his cell phone. It took effort and immense concentration to remember how to make a call. No answer. I was distraught and momentarily paralyzed at what to do next. I thought Alan's phone was surgically attached to him! My mind was in slow motion. I had to talk to them in person. I couldn't leave a message about this. I considered calling Glenn, his other brother. I didn't have his work number. I called his wife, Linda. She was not at home. I had her cell number. No answer. I could not reach one person in Callum's family. I panicked. I was torn between trying to talk to his family and rushing back into his room. I could hear him wheeze and gasp and wanted to be near him. I was anxious that I might not be there with him if he died. I wished for some magical person to help make these calls.

Linda and I used to work together in dispatch years before. I thought I remembered the work number and called there. She was not working, but they took a message and said they would try to get the message to her. She worked at the local police station. I felt confident they would succeed.

A few minutes later my cell phone rang. It was Linda.

"Lorna, I got the message that there is an emergency. What's wrong?"

I tried to fight back the tears as I answered.

"Callum has crashed and they said I should let family know. They don't know what is going to happen and it would be a good idea to have family come. I can't reach anyone. Mary, Walter, and Dorothy are at an Eastern Star meeting, and Alan isn't answering his phone. I have to get back into his room."

"I will get a hold of everyone. Don't worry. We will come to Saskatoon tonight," she assured me.

I felt an immense amount of relief and could regain a tiny sense of calmness that helped clear my mind. Knowing that everyone would be notified, I could again concentrate on what was happening to him.

I went back into Callum's room and saw him hooked up to a breathing machine. He was barely alert and quite sleepy. I didn't know if he understood what was going on. It was hard to talk to him because he was wearing an oxygen mask. I looked at him and tried hard to make myself believe he was going to get through this. I never felt more alone.

I remembered how I used to flippantly say, "We aren't that far away from anyone and we could get there quickly if there was an emergency." I learned it wasn't that easy.

That day, a few hours seemed like an eternity. I wanted someone with me. I needed someone with me that instant. That meant if I didn't want to wait for family, I had to ask for help. I started thinking of the people I knew in Saskatoon.

Most of our time spent in Saskatoon had revolved around cancer and the Cancer Centre. I made no friends outside of the ladies who worked in my office building. Both had evening programs and would be busy. They were great work friends and that was the extent of our friendships. I was uncomfortable asking them to step into this drama. There were two people who worked for Callum whom I felt comfortable having with me. I looked at my watch and saw it was after 4:30 p.m. and getting late to call anyone at their office. I decided to try anyway and called the *StarPhoenix* newspaper main line. I was hoping that maybe at least one of Callum's department managers, Wendy or James, might still be at work. Instantly, the call went into voice mail. I kicked myself for not putting their cell phone numbers in my phone contact list. I desperately hoped I had an email on my phone with a direct line for one of them.

I found an email with the number to Wendy's direct line. I was overcome with relief when she answered her phone. I did my best to tell her what was happening and asked if she could come and stay with me for a while.

"I'll be there in about a half hour," she reassured me. "I can stay for a little while. I will call James, and see if he can come and stay when I have to leave."

"Thank you so much," I said to Wendy. I was so thankful someone was coming. I couldn't imagine being there any longer without someone by my side.

That part wasn't over for me. While I waited for my troops to arrive, Dr. Haider said, "Come with me, let's go for a walk."

He put his arm around me for a brief moment. It wasn't going to be good news. We'd only had one appointment with Dr. Haider, and he was taking me away from the room where my husband was fighting for his life. The arm of comfort didn't stop the lump from forming in my throat and feeling like my heart had just dropped into my stomach. This couldn't be happening.

Suddenly, I felt even more alone, with the shield of armour trying to protect me.

"He has Acute Respiratory Distress Syndrome," he told me. "Does he want to be intubated? How far do we go with life saving actions, if we get there?"

My face must have told the story of how much I disbelieved what was happening.

Dr. Haider continued, "Do you understand what I am saying?"

I insisted that Callum deserved a chance. After all we had gone through we couldn't give in that quickly.

Dr. Haider kept saying, "As long as it's reversible. You want us to do everything, as long as it's reversible."

I had to ask, "When do we find out if it's reversible?"

“Within a few hours,” he said.

“Do everything you can,” I directed.

He nodded. “I really feel you made the right decision.”

It was then that I realized just how alone I was feeling and how desperately I wanted someone with me. Asking for this help when I was alone was hard for me. I tended to worry a lot about other people and tried to shield them from the “bad stuff.” I gave myself a lot of credit for knowing that this was a time to ask, and accept, help. My husband was lying in bed with a machine forcing air into his lungs so he could breathe. I tried to be prepared that he might not make it through the night. I didn’t want to be alone if it happened, and it would be a few hours yet before any family arrived. Thankfully, Wendy and James unselfishly helped me through those hours.

When I accepted help from others it gave them a chance to know they made a difference. I knew the satisfaction and appreciation I felt when I helped someone. I was thankful I found a way for others to have those wonderful feelings.

Many people helped us over the years. I’d love to write about each time those special people stepped up with offers of assistance. There were too many people who helped and too many stories to fit into this book. You know who you are. From help moving (many times) to being there through surgeries and scary times. It might have been an email, a phone call, a letter, or a great joke. All of it made a difference to us and helped Callum fight for as long as he could. You made my life easier. I suspect there were times I had help and didn't realize it was happening! Thank you, each and every one.

There is no exercise better for the heart than reaching down and lifting people up.

~ John Holmes, poet

REFLECTION

The indisputable lesson is that when you are a caregiver, you can't do it alone. Every second of help you get makes a difference. It could be a meal, a visit, or buying groceries—ask for what you need. People are waiting to help. Give them a job!

TIPS

1. Make a list of everything you need help with. Include driving to appointments, picking up medication, groceries, pre-cooked meals, lawn cutting, snow shovelling. Whatever you need. When someone asks how they can help, let them pick something off the list. You can also use www.lotsahelpinghands.com to schedule your needs. It was a big help to me.
2. When you have friends/family staying with you, be specific about what you need. They want to know how to help. Once we were clear with our visitors that they were in charge of meals, they were happy to do it. Being specific was essential to peace in the home!
3. Have a list of contact numbers for anyone you might need to call on for help. Keep the list in your contacts on your phone, computer, and a hard copy somewhere at home.

TIME FOR YOUR REFLECTION

1. What does it feel like to ask for and receive help?

2. What stops you from asking for, and accepting, help?

3. What are some ways you can empower your loved one to ask for help?

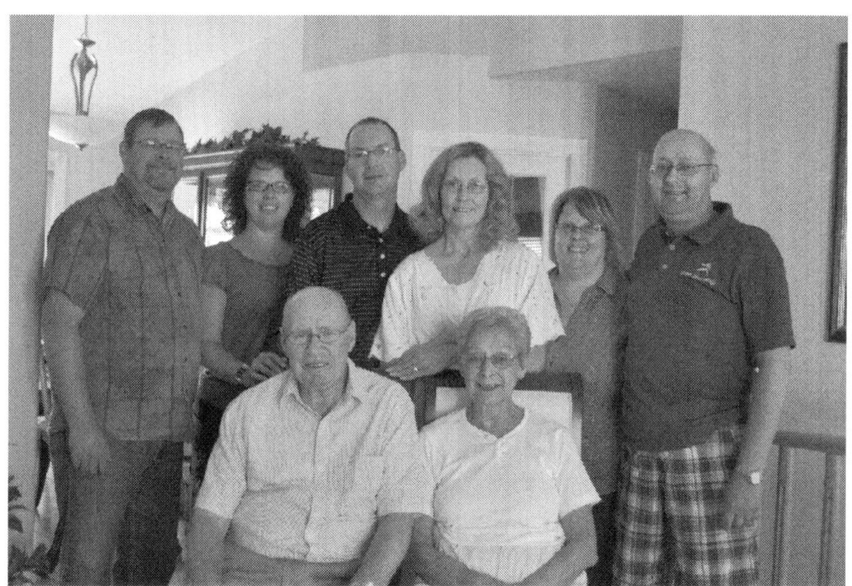

Back row: Glenn, Linda, Alan, Dorothy, Lorna, Callum
Front Row: Walter, Mary (Callum's parents)

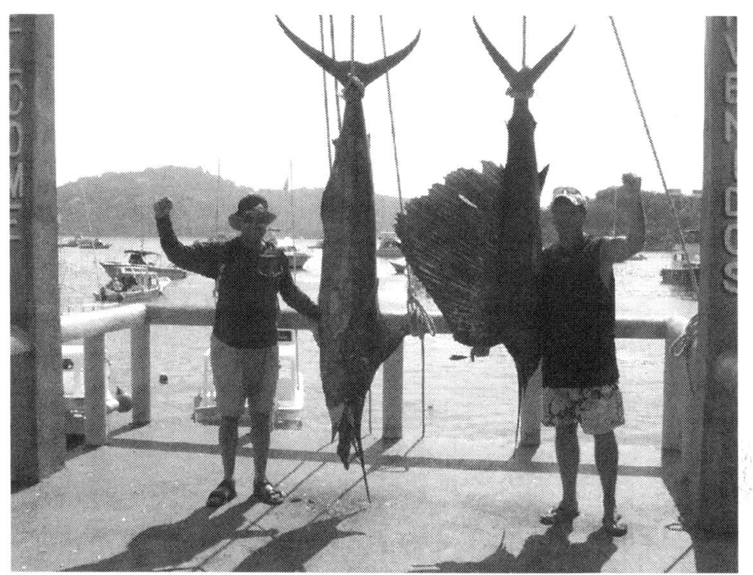

Deep sea fishing, Ixtapa 2008

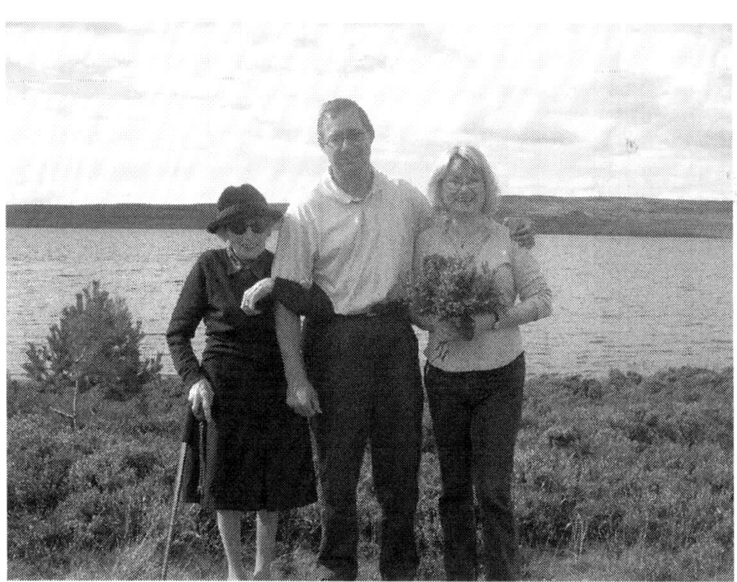

Callum with Nana Campbell & Aunt Fiona, Scotland 2006

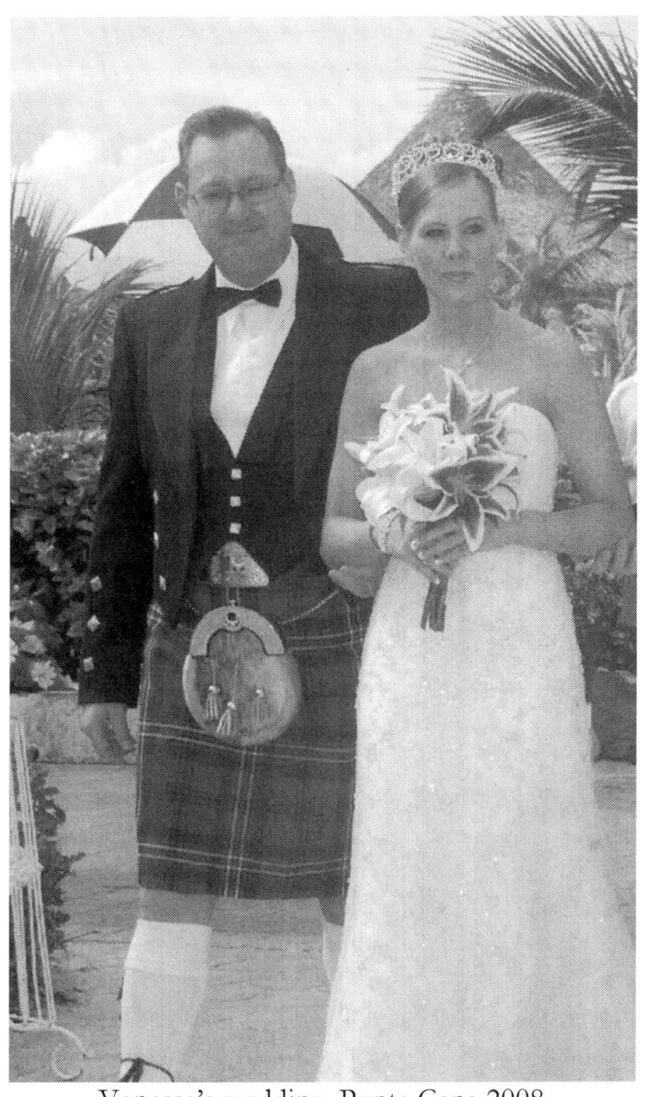

Vanessa's wedding, Punta Cana 2008

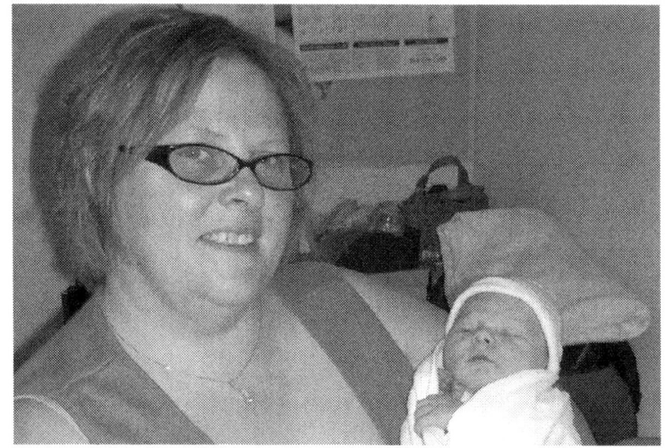

Loving Grandma and Cade, July 2009

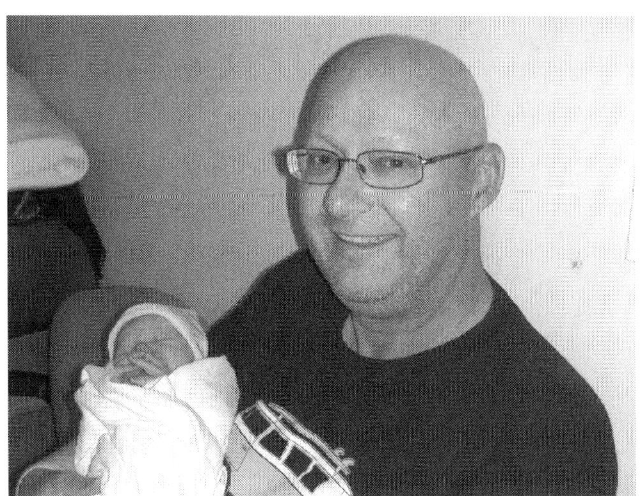

Proud Grandad and Cade, July 2009

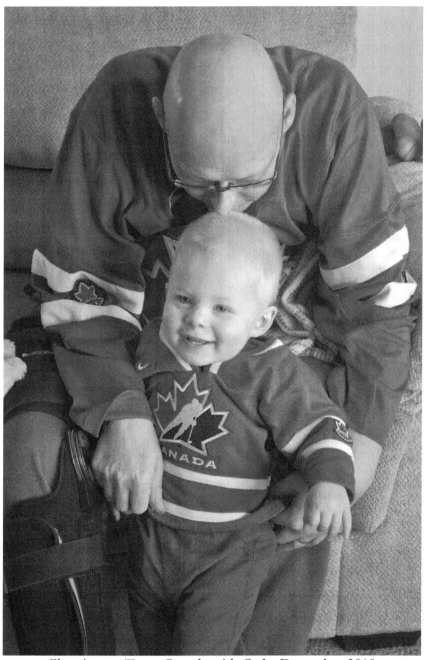

Cheering on Team Canada with Cade, December 2010

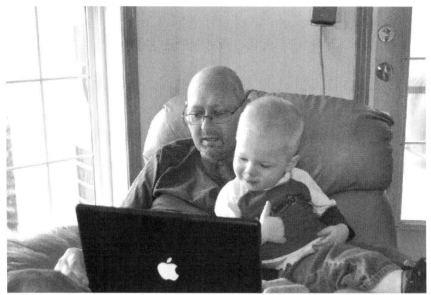

Grandad and Cade on Skype with great-grandparents

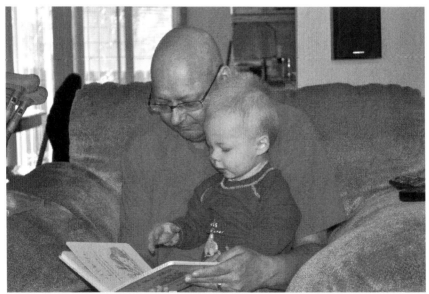

Grandad and Cade enjoying a book

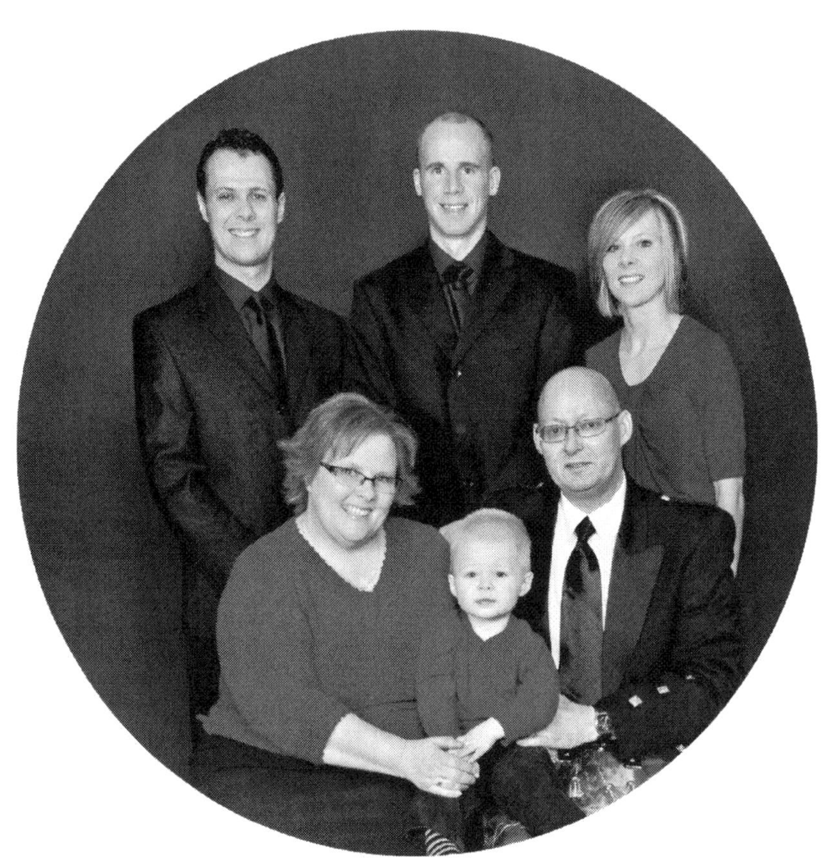

The Scott Clan, January 2011

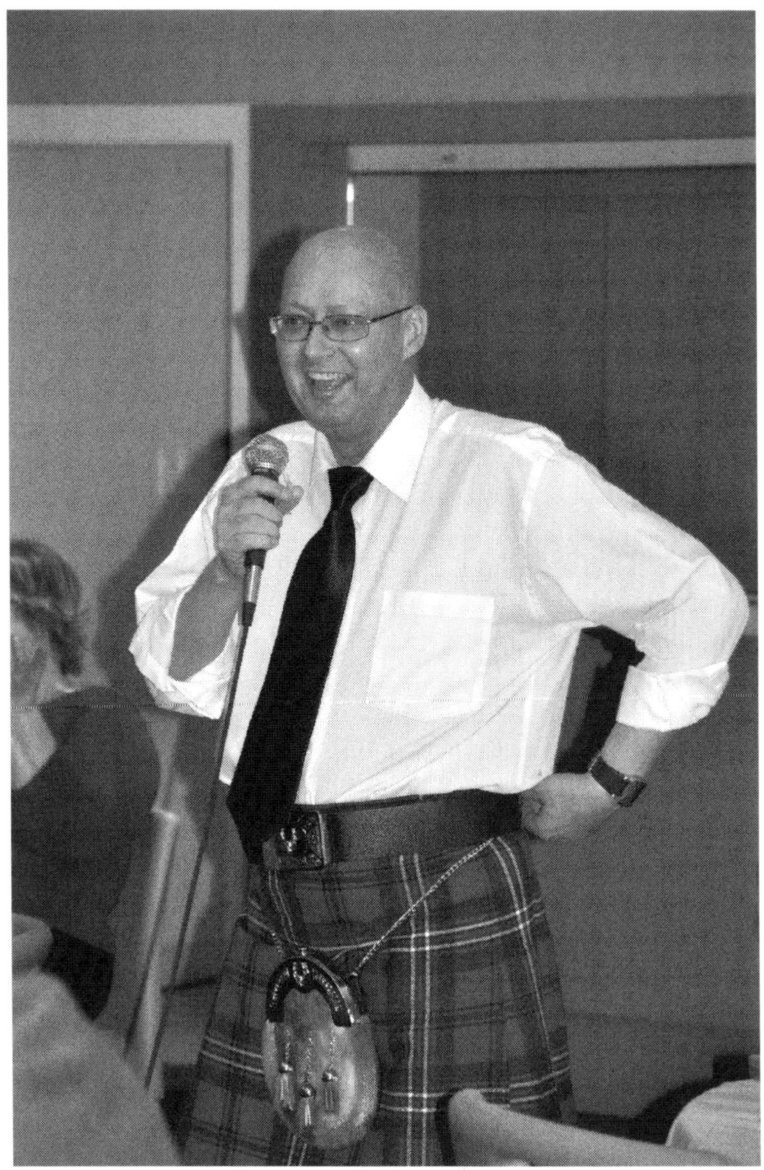

Giving thanks for a wonderful 50th birthday celebration

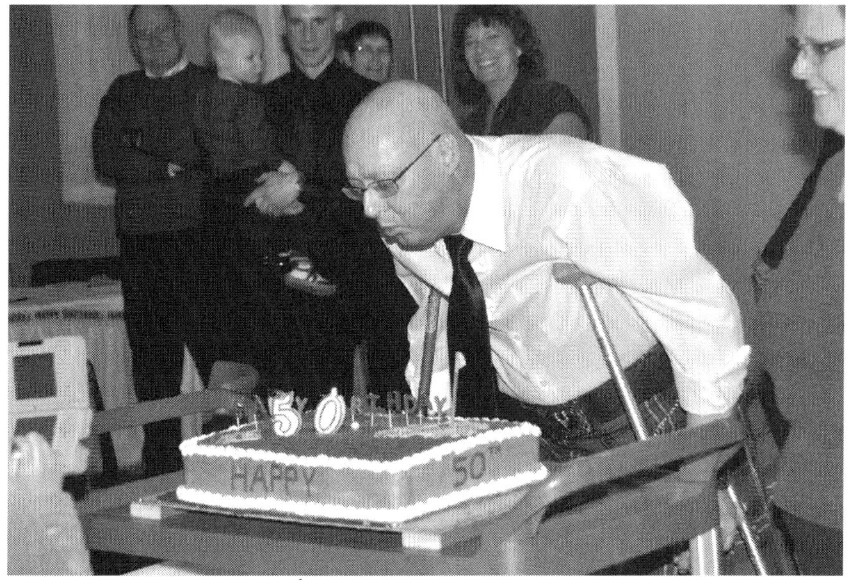

50th birthday, January 2011

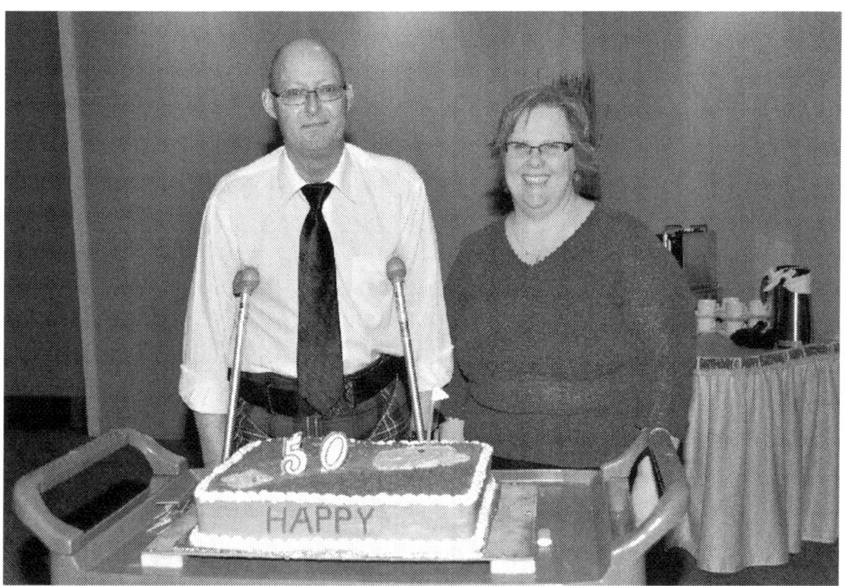

50th birthday, January 2011

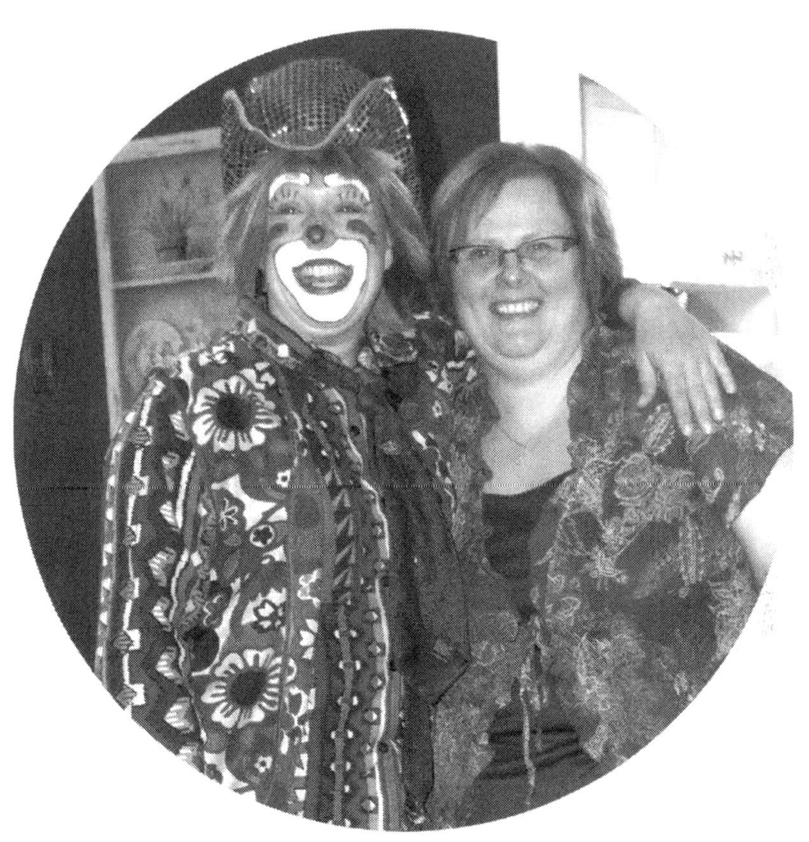

Lorna's 50th birthday & the birthday clown

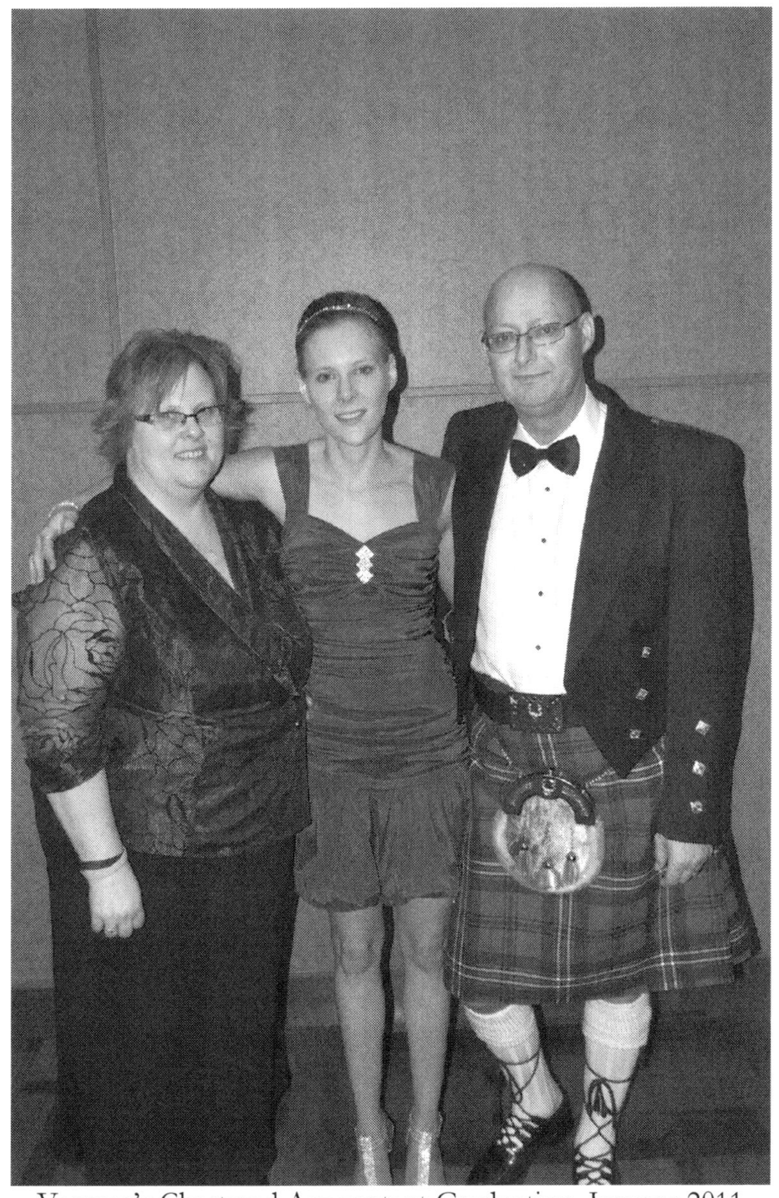

Vanessa's Chartered Accountant Graduation, January 2011

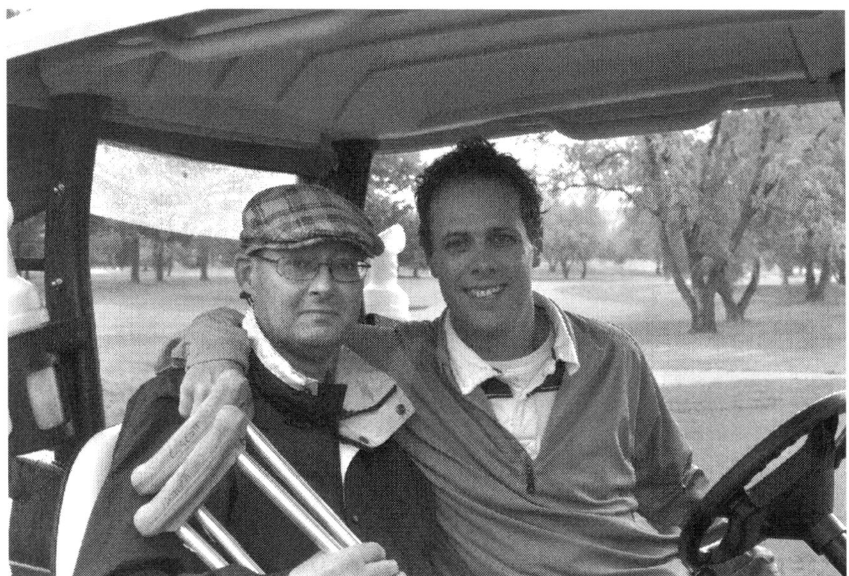

Victoria Day Classic, 2011

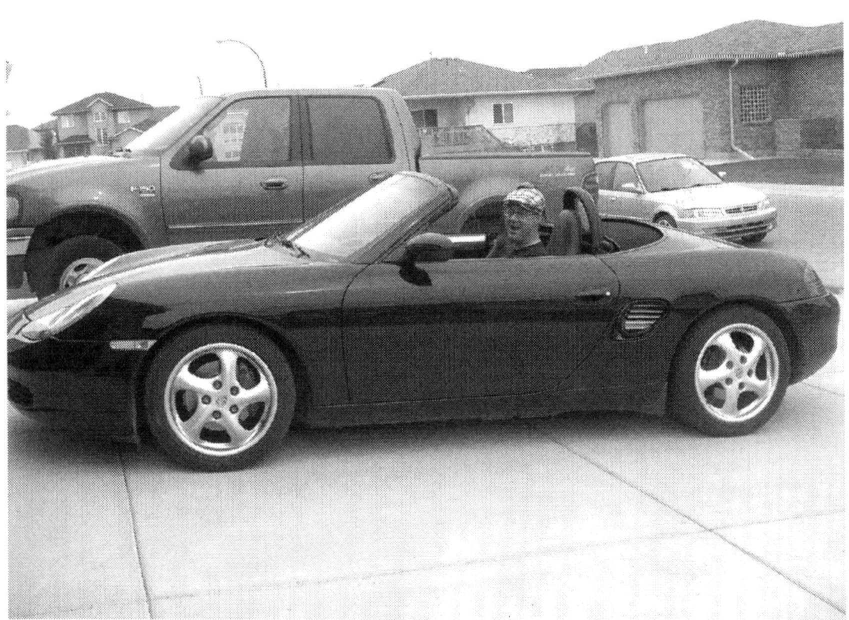

The car of his dreams, 2000 Porsche Boxster, June 2009

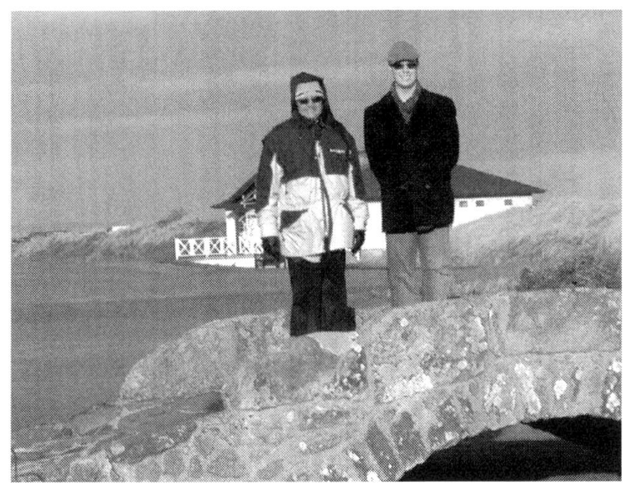

At the birthplace of golf, Swilcan Bridge
at St. Andrews Golf Course, January 2009

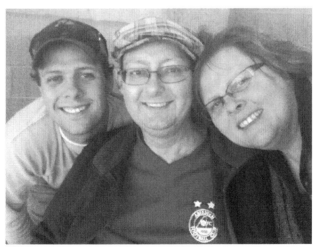

Callum, Lorna and Jamie, U2 Concert, June 2011

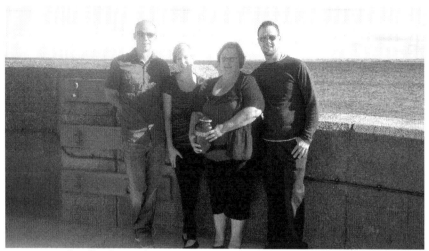

The final good-bye: Lorna, Jamie, Vanessa & Stuart,
Fraserburgh, Scotland, September 2013

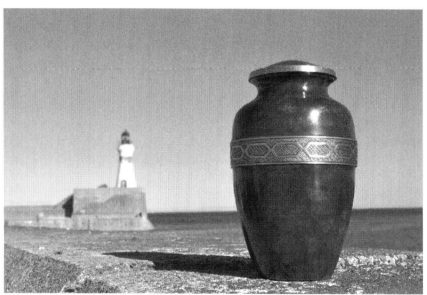

Callum returns home, to where it all began

Chapter Eight

Taking Care Of Myself

Our bodies are our gardens to which our wills are gardeners.

~ William Shakespeare, English poet and playwright.

Learning to take care of myself was one of my greatest challenges during those caregiving years. "Take care of yourself," the girls at work would say. "Remember to look after you!" my family said with concern.

Great advice. It made sense and was really important. What I really needed was for someone else to look after me. From the initial moment of hearing the dreadful news, I put myself on the back burner and focused on Callum's needs. I let his health trump mine. I had enough to deal with trying to come to terms with my husband having Stage 3C colorectal cancer. I had no idea how to fit taking care of me into an already overwhelming schedule. I didn't know where to start. The stress was something I had never experienced. The powerlessness was more than I could bear. The overwhelming combination of these two things crushed any attempt to look after my own needs.

Looking back, I realize there were three phases to my self-care and coping strategies: phase one after the initial diagnosis; phase two after Callum was diagnosed with terminal cancer; and phase three during the last six months that he was alive.

His first cancer treatment lasted only a few months, and I managed to get through it with few consequences from lack of self-care. I had the emotional and practical support of family and friends. They helped prepare healthy meals and provided good old-fashioned listening. After the initial treatment and before the terminal diagnosis, I was able to make a shift and put some focus on looking after me.

I liked having the time to pay attention to my health, physically and emotionally. I rejoined Curves and became a regular, three to four times a week, workout girl. I loved seeing my body get toned and my muscles get strong. I usually went with a friend so it was a social and fun time. Weight loss had been a long time battle and the Curves eating plan helped me get back on track and lose some weight. I got more fit, lost weight, and overall felt great.

What helped me stay committed to these self-care necessities was doing the workouts right after work and diligently planning meals and grocery lists. After Callum's surgery was over, and we reclaimed our normal activities, it became easier to incorporate these things into my schedule. I added to my self-care regimen regular appointments with my massage therapist, chiropractor, and numerous hours in the infrared sauna. Regular golf in the summer was not only a physical activity—it also gave me some emotional and mental stress relief.

Things changed after we moved to Saskatoon. That is when phase two began. I decided to find a Curves fitness centre. In the past, it was the one fitness centre I committed to the most. I decided to try the one closest to the apartment where we were living. It was not the same. It was missing the energetic and friendly Red Deer staff who would pump me up.

Exercise at Curves is done on a circuit, and you move from machine to rest station to machine, spending thirty seconds on each one. In February 2008, I was making my way around the circuit. I followed a very nice lady about the same age as me. She was friendly, and it was easy to strike up a conversation with her. She had lost her husband to cancer about a year prior. She told me about some of their bad experiences at the Saskatoon Cancer Centre and with one oncologist in particular. This poor lady was so sad and bitter, still grieving her husband. I knew I didn't want to follow that path. I hoped it wouldn't happen to me.

They were friendly enough at the Saskatoon Curves. Yet, I missed the camaraderie we had at the Red Deer Curves. I never returned to the Saskatoon Curves. Perhaps it was all the extra things that needed to be done, like finding a place to live, getting ready to move, medical appointments in Calgary, and planning for a wedding reception, or maybe it was the conversation with the woman. I didn't feel comfortable there, and I didn't seem to fit it into my schedule. The habit was broken, which made doing anything like that even more difficult.

After the cancer had spread and the disease was terminal, I didn't know where I was supposed to find time or energy to take care of myself. At least not the way others thought I should be doing. Certainly not the way the experts recommended. Eat right, exercise, reduce your stress. All were very good suggestions. The problem wasn't that I didn't know what to do. It was that I didn't know how to make it happen or when to do it. I was great at organizing all the other parts of our lives, like medical appointments, groceries, working, laundry, and scheduling visits. When it came to me, I ran out of time, energy, and concentration. What I didn't run out of was guilt.

There was a little voice that would tell me life wasn't fair. For either of us. Over the course of the two years after Callum went on long-term leave, he became more and more housebound. When I wasn't at work, I had no desire to leave the house unless absolutely necessary. Most often there were not enough hours in my day to keep up with work, appointments, and daily household chores, let alone fit in any social time. Still, I felt guilty that I had work to give me a chance to get away from the four walls of our house. I had connections with people. I laughed. I felt useful. Callum lost all of that when he was no longer working.

I found different ways of coping with stress. Some of it would fall into the self-care category. Some of it wouldn't. My soul was most in need of nurturing, so I spent hours on the computer searching for positive quotes and websites with positive and uplifting messages. Anything that could give me back some of my power. I also spent hours on the computer looking for information about colorectal cancer, clinical trials, and new research. I found support from the Colorectal Cancer Association of Canada (CCAC) and the LIVESTRONG™ Foundation.

The LIVESTRONG™ Foundation offered many types of assistance. I became a LIVESTRONG™ grassroots community volunteer in Saskatoon to help raise awareness of local cancer issues. This was empowering for me and I felt like I could do something that would make a difference. I took advantage of their counselling services for caregivers and access to clinical trial information. I would often browse their website for support issues and suggestions on what to ask the doctors. When they launched the livestrong.org website for supporting healthy lifestyle and cancer prevention, there was something that directly related to my self-care.

I found an enormous amount of emotional, practical, and research support from the CCAC. My initial inquiry to the organization led me to their lead researcher, Filomena Servidad-Italiano. Both of her parents passed away from colon cancer, and she was passionate about making lives better for those diagnosed with colorectal cancer. The association was based in Eastern Canada and was more aware of many new treatment options and clinical trials available in the eastern United States. She offered to include me in the email list for the support group she co-facilitated. This gave me access to monthly updates on patients and information on the latest research for nutrition, drug treatments, surgical treatments, and clinical trials. Fil became my go-to person whenever I had questions about treatment plans and sides effects. With her support and encouragement, I was most confident whenever I was advocating on Callum's behalf.

Being positive and looking for alternatives were great coping mechanisms. I found I felt better about myself and had comfort knowing that I did everything I could to help Callum fight the disease. The problem was that it meant I was sitting and looking at a computer for hours. I did that at work and then did it at home. It seemed a lot easier to do that than to get my butt off the chair and go for a walk. The research and inspiration I found surfing on the computer became a priority. I liked to use the excuse that I didn't want to leave him alone, especially when he no longer worked and was home all day by himself. I tried to get him out to walk so he could have the benefits of exercise. He couldn't walk fast or far. That idea didn't last long.

By October 2008, Callum was just finishing whole brain radiation and restarting regular chemotherapy treatments. I was finding it difficult to find the time or desire to organize myself to do any physical activity out of the house. It would be good for both of us to be more active, so I decided we would buy a treadmill. Both of us could use it and once he was home all the time, he could break up his activity into five or ten minute increments, whatever he could handle.

Callum tried using the treadmill. He was quite apprehensive because he had numbness in his feet from the chemo drug and was afraid he would get hurt. I couldn't blame him for not using it. I put the treadmill right behind the couch so I could watch television while I walked. It worked for a while. It didn't take much to knock me off track, though. It could be weekend visitors. It could be that I had long hours either at work or at the hospital, or both. Working on fitness became a stumbling block for me. I never seemed to exercise steady enough to get over that hump and reach the point where I had more energy. Many days I was just too damn tired and just didn't care.

I remember it seemed to be too complicated. I wouldn't have the right clothes on, which meant I would have to go find some. I wondered what the temperature was like in the basement and would I need long sleeves or short sleeves. I had to find my runners. I would have to find something on the television, or my Mp3 player. On a regular day in a regular life I would do these things without thinking. With all that was going on keeping things straight with Callum, I didn't want to make one more decision. My brain was tired. The thoughts came slowly and were often very deliberate in their pace. By the time I managed to get through all these obstacles, I was too tired and either I'd go on the computer or go to bed and watch some television. Walking on a treadmill was too hard to organize.

There was a direct correlation between the stability of my life and the regularity of my physical activity. There were days, especially once Callum was using a wheelchair regularly, that I felt like I had lots of exercise. I realize now that I confused exercise with being busy. I had lots to do and was in motion a lot. Not much of that gave me the benefits of good exercise.

Generally, the attention I gave to my diet kept me nourished. I have battled weight issues for years and had learned many different theories on healthy eating. I incorporated many of them into my daily eating habits. Callum had pretty good eating habits. His weaknesses were carbohydrates and red meat. He did most of the cooking so I would go along with whatever he cooked. One of his favourite comfort foods was mince and tatties. For those on the North American side of the pond, that is hamburger stew and boiled potatoes, fluffed but not mashed. I decided the best I could do was make as many good eating choices as possible, and to not berate myself when I didn't. I also needed my own comfort food. The weight loss experts might disagree, but when my world was falling apart, a few minutes with a chocolate dipped, soft serve ice cream cone gave me some pleasure. Yes, it was short lived. When it came to pleasure, I took what I could get.

I leaned toward what some people call complementary or alternative medicine for self-care. For a number of years before Callum was diagnosed, I had regular chiropractic treatment. When we moved to Red Deer, I was referred to an amazing chiropractor, Dr. Darren. The best thing about his clinic was that there was a holistic philosophy to it. He hired clinical massage therapists and expanded the upper floor into a spa. The spa had a hairdresser, relaxation massage, and aesthetician services. I enjoyed many pampered days at the clinic and spa. I took advantage of the pampering so much that they started letting me use the staff stairway from the sauna upstairs to the chiro treatment room downstairs. They became a family to me.

I found benefits to all of these treatments. I liked the massage to keep my muscles loose. My shoulders would get so tight I thought I was a masochist to go through some of the deep tissue massage treatments! I recommended they find some kind of a treatment where I could leave my shoulder muscles at the clinic and exchange them for ones that weren't as tight. We never did find a way to make that work.

Chiropractic treatments kept my spine aligned. I didn't have the most ergonomically correct workspace at my office and golf usually pushed and pulled the spine around. I used to struggle with keeping a good maintenance schedule with chiropractic and massage and found one thing that really helped was making the next appointment when I was paying for the one I just had.

The infrared sauna was priceless. This type of sauna has been used in Eastern medicine for years. I usually stopped in to use the sauna a minimum of twice a week, and most often three times. The published benefits were helping to boost the immune system, increasing blood circulation and burning calories, among many others. I loved it, regardless of what it did. I would often feel like I had just spent twenty-five minutes at the beach. I always felt better after a session. It might have been the fact that I was 100% alone for twenty-five minutes. No phone calls, no staff, no email. That alone made it all worthwhile.

I enjoyed the sauna so much I bought one after we moved to Saskatoon. I read some research had that suggested there might be a correlation between keeping the body warm and slowing down the growth of cancer cells. Callum had heard me rave so much about the sauna for more than two years that he started to use the sauna too. I think that was his chance to have some thinking space and solitude.

The effects of not having regular exercise and not paying attention to proper eating were obvious. Any weight I lost while in Red Deer was slowly regained. That left me having less energy and making it more difficult to take over some of the more physical household duties once Callum couldn't do them anymore. This also affected my sleep. I started to have trouble falling asleep and would wake up in the middle of the night and not be able to go back to sleep. I was reluctant to take sleeping pills. I didn't like taking medication. Someone suggested instead of sleeping pills I should take melatonin. I tried it and it seemed to work quite well. I used it quite regularly until I heard on The Doctors TV show that it was not regulated in North America so there was no way to know for sure whether or not I was getting the right dose. In Europe, it was given by prescription. I decided I wasn't willing to mess around with it on a regular basis anymore.

When I went on short-term disability in the months before Callum passed away, I had to see a psychiatrist to satisfy insurance requirements. He prescribed some sleeping pills and I gave in and started using them. I learned to make sure I took them before I went to bed and not after lying awake for an hour or more. I didn't feel groggy in the morning as long as I had about seven hours sleep. If Callum was sick or there might be a reason I'd have to wake up during the night, I wouldn't use them. They helped me go into a real deep sleep. I learned that I liked to have a good night's sleep more than I wanted to avoid medication.

I had been diagnosed with high blood pressure in 2002 and was on medication ever since. The good part about that is that wherever we lived I had to find a doctor right away. That is one thing I did faithfully. I never wavered from my blood pressure medication, and I made sure I kept those appointments.

One thing I really missed in Saskatoon was having a friend. Callum and I learned to really like each other's company, but this was the first time we had barely any social time outside of work. There was little time or energy for us to make friends. He spent at least half the time sick from the side effects of chemotherapy and radiation. I worked, cared for him when necessary, and took on more and more responsibility as he grew sicker.

The "ladies who lunched" saved my sanity many days. I was a real social being, and I needed to spend time with people. These ladies all worked in the same building as I did. There was Linda, Lorna (not me, a different one!), and Laney. Laney's name was really Elaine but to be a lady who lunched you needed an "L" name to join Lorna, Linda and Lorna. There was no particular regular day for lunch. Sometimes it was a spur of the moment idea. Other times we'd organize a day and time that everyone was available. It was usually every couple of weeks and was a nice chance to get away from the office and chat. Many times our conversation was not related to work and that was even better. These brief moments gave me a look into what it was like to have a regular life, with regular worries. I could escape from my world of despair and imagine that my life was normal.

By the time we moved back to Medicine Hat in 2011, Callum was very sick and I had really lost sight of any of my needs. I moved into phase three of self-care. I was in survival mode. I did what had to be done. My doctor encouraged me to get out and walk. He said it would relieve some stress and I would sleep better. He told me it would help me feel better. This information was not new to me. It was hard to get moving. I was exhausted from poor sleep and immense stress. Trying to move my body wasn't easy. My sister, Val, tried her best to get me out walking. We did get out a few times. It was nice and I did feel better. For a couple of weeks, we kept it up. It became a challenge to squeeze in the time when we were spending half the night at the emergency room and more than six hours a day at the hospital for blood transfusions.

As Callum's health became increasingly unpredictable, I was reluctant to do anything away from the condo building. There was still a solution. The condo complex had an indoor pool. Val loved the water so she managed to get me in the pool a few times too. Some days the water was cold so we did a few aquacise moves and warmed up in the hot tub. I appreciated having someone look after me even though it felt foreign and uncomfortable. I felt relieved after I was out of the apartment and no longer had to pay attention to what was going on with him, I was still too wound up to really let go and relax. I soaked in the silence of the pool area and sought out as much peace and calm as possible. When I had little motivation and desire for anything, having someone set a time to come and take me out really helped.

The best example of the state of my ability to look after myself in those last few weeks was that I didn't see anything wrong with setting an alarm every hour to hour and a half through the night so I could check on

Callum. I didn't see how interrupting my sleep affected my body and my mind. He wasn't going out much so our days were pretty quiet. I just figured I could have a nap and everything would be better. I had no idea I had lost the ability to rationally think things through.

My body took on the brunt of my stress when I was focused on caregiving. After Callum passed away, the first change I noticed was how much sleep I needed. For a few months I slept. A lot. There were many nights I slept more than twelve hours. There were many days if I slept less than twelve hours I would have to have a nap in the afternoon.

The less obvious effects showed up later. When I settled into living in Medicine Hat, I started to see a new massage therapist. I soon realized she was brought into my life to help me heal in all ways. When I walked into the room, she instantly knew what was going on with me and would add emotional and spiritual healing to the massage. It was like we had been connected for years.

One of the first things she noticed was that my jaw and the muscles around it were extremely tight. She said I must have been clenching for quite a while. She massaged outside my face and neck and inside my mouth. Slowly, the muscles started releasing. About a year after Callum passed away I was standing in the kitchen and I heard a pop. Suddenly I could open my mouth really wide. My jaw finally released. Until then I hadn't realized it was so tight. I could now open my mouth wide enough to bite a sandwich properly. I didn't talk funny any more. I finally played my flute properly. I thought I was just out of practice the year before. I couldn't play properly because I couldn't open my mouth. I had no idea when the clenching started, and was glad it was over.

Another piece of hidden evidence that I hadn't handled the stress well was when one of my teeth broke. When I went to have it fixed, the dentist mentioned there were two or three more teeth showing signs of cracking. These hadn't shown up in the last x-rays taken at the office of my dentist in Saskatoon. I was sure they were cracking because of the intense clenching I was doing.

My self-care routines over the six years definitely depended on the intensity of Callum's health issues. Having a workout buddy in Red Deer helped me stay in an exercise routine. I can't help but wonder if I had been able to build some friendships and found a workout buddy in Saskatoon if things might have been different. I had a gap between knowledge and action. I used to work with women and families and encourage self-care. I knew the importance of self-care. I knew many different ways to look after myself. Most days I ran out of time doing other things before I worried about me. If I had taken the time, and made the commitment to myself, I could have made some changes in my routine most days. It was easier not to bother.

Don't sacrifice yourself too much, because if you sacrifice too much there's nothing else you can give and nobody will care for you.

~ Karl Lagerfeld, fashion designer

REFLECTION

It has been a journey trying to get through all the layers of self-care now. I worry about how much damage the constant high level of stress has caused my body on the inside. I have worried that it might increase my risk for cancer. At the time, the most important thing to me was that I cared for Callum. As long as I could do that, I put little effort into looking after me. It was the bare minimum and missed the mark. In a perfect world, I wouldn't have sacrificed my self-care for anything. Making my health and sanity a priority would have helped me look after Callum even better. I would have been able to give myself the love and care I deserved and desperately needed. I was a caregiver who needed a caregiver.

TIPS

1. Change your mindset by meditating daily and repeating positive affirmations. Whenever the fears show up, focus on the present. You can say things like, "I am having a peaceful and happy day" or "I can handle anything thrown my way."
2. Find a reliable and compassionate workout buddy to help you keep doing some physical activity.

3. Seek social support from friends and family. Find someone to confide in, someone to take you for coffee, play games, go to a movie, or chat.

TIME FOR YOUR REFLECTION

1. What self-care activities have you enjoyed in the past and which ones are you doing right now?
2. What are some ways you are neglecting yourself? What are the consequences if you don't look after yourself?
3. How does it feel to take time for you? Do you deserve it?

Chapter Nine

Gratitude

Gratitude is an art of painting an adversity into a lovely picture.

~ Kak Sri

When my world was falling apart, I found solace in gratitude. Stepping into gratitude really helped me shift from despair and sadness to a state of joy. It might have seemed like an oxymoron to do that. It wasn't always easy. My life sucked. I never dreamed I'd be a caregiver. The reality was that life was for living, and hanging out in the darkness of despair was not living. I learned to be creative and find different perspectives in order to see what I could be grateful for. For six years, I bounced back and forth between wishing and hoping things would be different, to accepting how it really was and finding gratitude for what I did have in my life.

I was extremely grateful for the love and support of family and friends. I was surprised at the genuine caring shown by so many people and humbled by the number of friends and acquaintances who requested to be included on the email update list. I had no idea how many lives Callum and I touched until so many people were interested in following our journey and supporting us. Even more profound for me were the replies, sometimes from people I barely knew, that were full of compassion, empathy, support, and love. I may not have known them well, but each of them had been impacted by their relationship with Callum or me. It was a less lonely place knowing there was global support in our corner.

Often, it was smack in the middle of a dark time that brought the deepest gratitude. Callum and I seldom shared a lot about each other's work lives. There were occasional chats here and there over dinner. Usually it was nothing more than to answer the question, "How was your day?"

Somehow the idea that work was work, and home was home, just fell into place. The sneak peek I had into Callum's relationship with work and the relationship with his colleagues happened when we started moving from city to city. The people who worked for and with him were always immensely sad to see him leave. These sneak peeks were only the tip of the iceberg for what I would come to learn about the depth of the respect and admiration his staff and colleagues had for him. The true understanding happened when he went on long-term disability.

Life changed dramatically for both of us when Callum was told he could no longer drive because of the brain tumours. He lost his independence and I gained more responsibility. I was now the only driver in the house. Since he could also no longer drive, I took him to his office on the day he informed his staff of this latest development.

His office was large with a beautiful maple wood desk, stained black, with matching credenza and hutch. In the corner was a round table with four chairs. I chuckled inside when I noticed the plastic replicas of the Dilbert cartoon strip characters on the top of his hutch. That is the humour he enjoyed. I took notice of the pictures of the two of us and the children on his desk. Everything he loved about his career tied directly to his passion—his family. There were newspapers laying around on the table and the desk. It was a typical office for the advertising manager of a daily newspaper.

I sat at the round table while Callum decided what to pack and what to leave. He wasn't a pack rat so there was very little to gather together. He stood behind his desk shuffling papers here and there. He was trying to collect his thoughts, and his courage to go to the staff meeting. He tried hard to have a poker face, but I could see his lip briefly quiver and he quickly composed himself. He didn't want to give any clues to what he was going to say at the staff meeting. The air became heavy with emotion. I could feel his anxiety, disappointment, and extreme sadness. Neither of us knew what to say so we sat there in silence.

I used to say he lived and breathed newspapers, and that his blood was likely black and white, not red. That was the day when he had to say good-bye to it. He hoped against hope that he would return. I wanted to believe he was right. I had to believe. It was the only way I knew how to support him. It was the only way he could cope.

Callum glanced at his watch. It was time. He walked over to me and I stood up, gave him a bear hug and a kiss.

With tears rolling down my cheeks, I said, "Good Luck!"

He gave me an extra hard squeeze and took a few deep breaths. Away he went to the meeting to announce he was going on a long-term leave. I knew he reassured them he was going to beat cancer and would return to work.

It seemed like an eternity before he was back. He walked into the office and I could tell by his red eyes that he'd let out some tears. That was the day I saw the "work" Callum.

The first thing he did was grab me and hold on with all his might. I stood there holding him as he cried. This was a man who wouldn't even hold hands in public. There we were, in his very public office, door open, and in an emotional embrace for all to see. What happened next really opened my eyes.

One by one, his staff came into the office. Some would try to remain stoic and shake his hand, say, "Good Luck," "Best Wishes," and "I'll miss you." Others bravely gave him a hug. Some cried. There were a few who were so upset they could not talk. Tears and hugs. That was all that was possible. Deep down, I believed everyone knew he wouldn't be back.

Being with Callum that morning was something for which I will always be grateful. I learned so much about him and his drive for success in the newspaper business. Most of all, I learned about his genius in the industry. I learned about the difference he made in the lives of those who worked for him. I learned how quickly he gained respect. And I learned how much he would be missed. I spent so much time in the past resenting his work because I thought it was his priority over our family. That morning in Saskatoon I found a way to embrace, physically and emotionally, Callum, the newspaper guy. My eyes and heart were opened, and I grew closer to being able to share that part of his life with him. I also came away knowing that I had to find a way to keep him connected to this world when he was on long-term leave. It was a piece of hope I wasn't willing to rip away from him.

When he was presented with an opportunity to move to Saskatoon and become the advertising director at the daily newspaper, it was a career move he had been dreaming about for years and would likely be the last step he'd take before he'd become a publisher. We took a risk when we moved to Saskatoon for him take on a new job when his health was unpredictable. He decided it was worth the risk. I was grateful he didn't hold back. He decided to follow his heart and his dreams. This was a deliberate and planned move.

We chose to move to Saskatoon because of the promises of a better future. I didn't know that there was also a bigger, unknown plan in place for us. Of all the places we lived, Saskatoon was the only city that had a fully operational cancer centre. Aside from the gamma knife treatments, he had access to all other treatment options and diagnostic tests only fifteen minutes from home. This turned out to be advantageous for me. It let me support him and continue working. When Callum could drive, he was able to get himself to and from many of his appointments, and I was close enough to take time from work to be with him for the rest. I underestimated the overall impact of the advantage of being in Saskatoon for the terminal part of his journey.

The Saskatoon Cancer Centre is a smaller agency, which made it easy for me to get to know everyone really well. I loved it when we arrived and they called us by name. I felt quite comfortable there and made personal relationships with oncologists, nurses, and clerks. That made my life easier. I learned whom I could trust and whom would most likely be able to answer my questions. I was included as an important part of the treatment team and equally to Callum. I was the main contact with the medical team. This took a lot of pressure off of him. He could focus on staying as healthy as possible. Our chosen path unexpectedly led us to the best place he could be for treatment of terminal cancer. My gratitude ran deep for how this turned out.

I am grateful he let me control as much as I did, especially with squeezing in our retirement and doing the things important to him. The monumental shift to fulfilling as many of his dreams as possible came after discovering The Passion Test®. This helped us live amazing lives for three years. I was grateful for learning this in time to make a difference for both of us.

Callum was a humble man and seldom asked for any grand desires. There were a few, though. One was taking our children to Scotland to introduce them to his family. We promised our children we'd take them when Vanessa was ten years old. She was twenty-six when we made the trip, only a few years behind schedule! He was still recovering from brain radiation and low on energy and stamina. We managed to make sure he had his rest and were able to do all the visiting we wanted to fit in. One particular day, Callum and Jamie's lives were changed forever. I am grateful the opportunity came, and that he was able to see what a wonderful son he had.

January 8, 2009 was Jamie's twenty-ninth birthday. We were staying in Fraserburgh with Callum's cousins, Peter and Sheena. Callum, Peter, and Jamie shared a deep love for the game of golf. Peter planned an extra special surprise for Callum, a trip to Carnoustie Golf Course and to the birthplace of golf—St. Andrew's. It was a family day and before sunrise seven of us, Peter and Sheena, Stuart and Vanessa, Jamie, Callum, and I all piled into the rented van and were on our way. It was January and too chilly to play so we enjoyed walking parts of both courses. The highlight of the day was having photos taken on the Swilcan Bridge at St. Andrews. It was a wonderful family day full of memorable moments.

Jamie knew going to the birthplace of golf with his dad would be a very special memory for him. This was accentuated with the knowledge that Callum would most likely not live another six months.

The depth of emotion Jamie felt was expressed in an email he wrote on the way back to Fraserburgh.

Wrote this on the way in from St. Andrews today. I wasn't going to post but I told myself if I did something like this I'd share it, so here it is. It's a little sappy, and much self-serving, so if that don't interest you then feel free to move along . . .

Birthday wishes

I wish I wasn't so old.

I wish you were here.

I wish I have a birthday as good as this again.

I wish health for my sister and her husband and future family.

I wish I would have come here sooner.

I wish for my dad to see my next birthday.

I wish to play golf with my dad at the places I saw today.

I wish I could stay here.

I wish everything I have for all of you.

I know so many who are not in touch with their siblings, parents, and cousins. I am so very fortunate for the family I have. I wish you could feel the love that I feel.

I wish my mom didn't have so much to worry for.

I wish for my dad to see my family, when it comes.

I wish you all knew how much I care for you all.

I wish I could see Peter and Sheena more.

I wish it was Saturday night.

I wish my family knew how important they are to me. I wish I reflected more of what they have instilled in me. I wish for the future that I will.

I wish I met Great-Nana sooner. I wish she could see me, and not just the colour of my shirt. I hope I live my life in a way that would make her proud.

I wish those two pints didn't go through me so fast, and that this drive was over.

I wish the world was a better place.

I wish we all got twelve weeks of holidays. We all deserve it, in my opinion.

I wish we put as much emphasis on the happiness of our brothers and sisters and we did the bottom line. The world would be a much better place then, and we'd all be happier and healthier.

I wish I had courage.

I wish, should it happen, then my dad will pass with pride of me.

I wish for him to be here for a long time, so I can make sure that happens.

I wish my dad knew how proud I am of him.

I wish to be half the man my dad is.

I wish I could be the sick one. I wish I could take the pain, and have it myself. For Dad and Mom both.

I wish every birthday was like this.

I wish I wasn't so stupid sometimes.

I wish for today to never end.

I wish I'd have shown better judgment in the past.

I wish I could give days like today to the people who gave today to me.

I wish so many people didn't worry about me.

But I'm glad that I have these people to do that.

I wish it was me that was sick. These people don't deserve this. Neither do I, I suppose, but I have less to lose, and I would gladly take it to ensure their health and prosperity.

I wish I had such moments of clarity when I was younger.

I wish every day was my 29th birthday.

The agony was evident and I was so proud that he bravely wrote from his heart, and courageously shared his pain with others.

Callum was tough on Jamie. He did it "for his own good." There were times I thought he was too harsh, and I learned when I read that blog that Jamie longed for acceptance from his dad. I was a middleman in their relationship.

He thought Jamie never listened to him, and Jamie felt like he would never live up to his dad's expectations. I knew different. I knew he only wanted his son to be the best he could be, and better than he ever was. I saw the Callum who wished he could take away Jamie's pain and help him to build a great life. I saw the man who also knew Jamie had to do it completely on his own.

I knew the Jamie who most wanted respect and love from his dad. I saw the Jamie who would do his best to be perfect and, like all of us, fall short and disappoint himself, and sometimes others. I saw the Jamie who tried to emulate his dad. I saw the Jamie who wanted to hear the words, "I'm proud of you, son. I love you."

Tears filled my eyes as I read about his pain. He bared himself for the world to see. Peter and his family told me how Jamie was hurting, thinking he was a big disappointment to his dad. Peter's daughter Kerri, who is the same age as Jamie, told me of Jamie crying in the back of the van as he was writing. I could no longer ignore this rift in their relationship. What was most important to me was that Callum would see and hear what Jamie so deeply felt that day.

He nearly cried as he learned the truth and depth of Jamie's emotions. This was a big lesson for him. He didn't realize the emotional shrapnel thrown in Jamie's path by the expectations he set for Jamie. This new awareness cut straight to his heart. The relationship between Callum and Jamie would never be the same. Thankfully, it was so much better.

In May 2011, a few short weeks before he passed away, Jamie won a major local golf tournament. He dedicated the win to his dad. Callum was there, supporting him as much as possible. And on that rainy day in May, he watched Jamie make a miraculous second shot—a great putt—and win the tournament. I was very grateful they found a way to love and respect each other so they could share the joy of the moment.

Callum deeply loved both of our children, more than they would ever know. Jamie tends to take after me and some of those traits irritated him. On top of the list would be the unique sense of time Jamie and I have, and the manner we organized our disorganization. He loved us anyway. Vanessa was the one he totally related to. She was a female "mini-me" of Callum. They shared logical thinking, patience, and planning. Neither were great risk takers. Their sameness sometimes elevated to a loud discussion, which was fun for Jamie and I to watch. One thing in their relationship that I was grateful for was that he not only lived to walk Vanessa down the aisle at her wedding, but he lived to see her reach her career goal. She was always "Daddy's little girl." Her career achievement was even sweeter because he was there. We were all grateful.

There is nothing I am more grateful for than Callum's determination and persistence to live. Especially when I wanted him to accept his fate and give in. As time went on, I found my gratitude was for things other people desperately feared. Continuing chemotherapy treatment, gamma knife brain radiation, and surgery to remove a brain tumour are things that frighten the strongest of the human race. For these, I was grateful.

After the terminal diagnosis my gratitude often centred around the medical issues. When the doctor would get the latest CT and MRI results and I heard that Callum would continue with chemotherapy, I was thankful. It meant that the cancer was still controlled and most likely we had another three months to make beautiful memories. It was not the life I chose but was the hand I was dealt. Brain radiation of any kind is terrifying. Gamma knife treatment holds one of the biggest spots of gratitude in my heart. The first treatment was successful in treating two tumours, and when one started growing again, the second treatment helped Callum live another eighteen months. My gratitude runs deep for this treatment. Brain surgery are two words nearly everyone would put on their "I don't want to hear" list. My gratitude for brain surgery is two-fold. First, he was determined to live every minute possible, and was brave enough to go through it. Second, we had more time with Callum. He lived to celebrate my fiftieth birthday party.

By the time he was nearing the end of his life, every day he woke up next to me was a great day. When we had the last oncologist visit on April 5, 2011 and found out that chemotherapy was no longer working, it was devastating. I refused to give into the darkness and strongly suggested we celebrate. I'd had enough tears and worry over the past five years that I didn't want to cry anymore. I wanted to celebrate Callum's courage. I wanted to celebrate his fight. I wanted to celebrate that he defied all odds and stumped the experts on his life expectancy. I wanted to celebrate that I could, we could, enjoy a very nice meal together. The cancer may have been raging inside of his body but I wasn't giving in. From the outside looking in it would appear that my life was shitty and I had no reason to have joy. Gratitude changes everything.

We can only be said to be alive in those moments when our hearts are conscious of our treasures.

~ Thornton Wilder, American playwright and novelist

REFLECTION

There was a long list of reasons for me to be resentful and angry. I did feel resentful and angry. I acted resentful and angry on many occasions. Once the temper tantrum was done I returned to gratitude. It was easy to be grateful for the good things in life. New jobs, getting a raise, having babies, getting married—all those life events bring gratitude. The challenge is to find gratitude when your life goes sideways. I don't know if any one moment is more deserving of gratitude than another. I do believe that gratitude is grounding. It brings comfort and peace. Gratitude isn't an illusion or magical. There is always something for which to be grateful. Don't get me wrong; I would change things in a heartbeat if it would bring Callum back. I planned to grow old and live to a ripe old age with him by my side. This is what I would have chosen if given the chance. I didn't get the chance. I adjusted my sails and became grateful for the life we did have. As Forest Gump said, "Life is like a box of chocolates. You never know what you're gonna get."

TIPS

1. Start a gratitude journal. Every day, write at least five things you are grateful for on that day.
2. Appreciation game: At the end of the day, take a few minutes to tell your loved one(s) what you appreciate about them. Have them do the same for you.
3. During the tough times, when it can be hard to find gratitude, set a timer for 2–3 minutes and do a "gratitude blast." In that length of time, write down everything you can think of that you are grateful for.

TIME FOR YOUR REFLECTION

1. What have you learned to be grateful for in your relationship with your loved one?
2. What are some ways you can show your gratitude to your loved one? To the medical team? To others?
3. What have you been the most angry or resentful about? What are one or two things you can find to be grateful about in that situation?

Chapter Ten

Saying Good-Bye

There are things that we don't want to happen but have to accept, things we don't want to know but have to learn, and people we can't live without but have to let go.

~ Team Lycans

When it came to how long Callum should live, he defied all odds, many times. It was no surprise when the medical professionals quit trying to predict exactly when he would pass away.

In fact, after the bone metastases were confirmed, Dr. Kundapar, the radiation oncologist, said, "He has long outlived any life expectancy we could have predicted."

He battled so many things during his fight with cancer that it was hard for me to believe one day he wouldn't win. Even though I lived through three years with Callum battling a terminal disease, knowing he was dying, when those final few days arrived it felt like he passed away too quickly. The last month with him was quite surreal.

I didn't want to see the many clues that the end was near. I was in my own protective bubble and liked it there. He was becoming weaker and more tired. Some days it took a lot of effort for him to continue eating and maintain a regular daily schedule. Once in a while he would get out of the apartment. The trips became fewer and fewer. I still believed it would be many months before I would lose him.

The first time his stoma bled was the first big clue that his fight was nearly over. He'd been having some minor bleeds and thought he was just bumping the stoma and making it bleed. On Saturday, June 11, 2011, it didn't just bleed. It was a hemorrhage. I was watching television and Callum had gone to the bathroom. He was slower moving by then, and I took no notice of how long he had been in the bathroom. When he came out of the bathroom he told me he had been bleeding and there had been quite a lot of blood. I had no idea how bad it really was because he diligently cleaned up the bathroom and his clothes. He was not going to let me know there was any emergency. I wouldn't let it go. I kept prodding and he finally told me there was enough blood to fill up two to three colostomy bags. After I figured out that he likely lost two to three cups of blood, I called an ambulance. That was trip number one to the emergency room.

The bleeding had stopped by the time the emergency room doctor examined Callum. He looked for the source of the bleed, stitched up some possible leaks and away we went home.

A few days later there was another bleed, worse than before. It wouldn't stop. Another ambulance. Another visit to the emergency room. This time the doctor tried to cauterize the leaks. There were so many. It looked like it was an arterial bleed because blood would squirt all over with just the slightest pressure on the stoma. There was talk of possible surgery, but it wouldn't happen that night. I wished they could find the problem and fix it.

With that much blood loss, blood transfusions became a necessity. I would take Callum to the lab for blood tests and up to the ward for the blood transfusion. There was no quick and easy way to do it. He was using a wheelchair whenever there was some distance to cover when we were out. He'd get himself into the wheelchair in the apartment. I'd push him through the door, down the hallway, and to the elevator. From the elevator, we wiggled through the two doors to the parking garage, to the car. He'd get himself into the car, and the wheelchair was put in the storage unit. When we arrived at the hospital, I would park, go into the hospital to get a wheelchair, back to the car to get Callum, and we'd go wheeling around the hospital. I quickly tired of this routine, but I had no choice, so I resigned myself to do what I had to do. Some days I resented having to do all of this for a mere five minutes in a lab to take blood. When I had the energy, I would seethe with anger that our lives were now like this. My life now revolved around him and his health problems—and while that had been the case for a number of years, the difference was now there was no bucket list to turn to. These miserable days were going to be the best we could hope for. Regardless of my own pity parties, I always had a lot of empathy for Callum. I knew how much he hated being dependent on me. I would get a second chance at life. He wouldn't.

I was worried about the unpredictability of the bleeds and I never wanted to leave him alone. There was no rhyme or reason to them. Sometimes they were controllable and other times it took time to get the bleeding under control. By the end of June, I spent most of my day, and night, waiting for the next bleed. At some level I knew this was not good. So did Callum. He decided it was time to have his family come so they could have their last conversations.

I fully and lovingly supported his decision. In the fog of seeing his health rapidly deteriorate and still hoping he'd get through this phase, these next steps helped me see reality. Every once in a while I needed a sharp reminder that he wasn't going to get through this. I accepted that we were in the final phase, and it was time to step into the role of gently assisting Callum with his last wishes. I set aside my pain to give my all to him for the time we had left. I had read about end of life care and had some ideas from what others had found helpful going through similar experiences. I knew we had a chance as a family for all to be at peace with Callum when he passed away. I genuinely wanted him to be at peace with his family. No regrets. My job was to help him set the stage for this to happen.

The condo complex where we lived had additional guest rooms we could use when we ran out of space in our own place. Mary and Walter slept in one of those rooms and spent the day with us in our condo. They stayed with us for over two weeks. During that time we had many visitors come and go. Jamie often stayed in our spare room, and Callum's brother and my parents used guest rooms when they were available.

Our condo was perfect for the two of us. It was a comfort to have so many people visit us. They helped with meals, groceries, and errands. Mary and Walter were by our sides the longest. They knew their way to the casino and would go there every once in a while so they could give us some privacy. I am sure they needed their privacy, too. I respected that these would be the last days they would spend with their son.

Trying to meet everyone's needs but my own became overwhelming. I yearned for a place where I could "just be." It was nowhere to be found.

I also started to fear that I was losing time to spend alone with Callum. Emotions ran through me like crazy. One night, as he was doing his bedtime ritual, I told him how I was feeling.

"I am glad they are here," I explained. "But I'm missing some of my alone time, and time with you."

The tears started flowing, and it became hard for me to talk.

"I'm afraid that if you don't wake up in the morning, I will have missed the chance to say what I need to say. I don't get enough time with just you." I cried as I choked back the tears.

He pulled me close to him and hugged me tight.

"I'll figure out something. Don't worry. We will have all the time we need," he said.

The crying released some energy and tension. I felt better after talking about this with Callum. I didn't know how he would make it better, but I knew he would. He worried about me so much. He wanted me to have peace.

"Let's go to bed and have a good cuddle," he said.

His reassurance calmed me down. I believed Callum would make sure we had more time for ourselves. I crawled into bed beside him. I rolled over, and he put his arm around me. I felt safe and secure. That lasted about three seconds.

"Oh no," Callum exclaimed.

I bolted up and looked at him, seeing the panic in his eyes.

"I'm going to bleed!" he said with urgency and a sense of fear.

So much for staying calm. I tried to help as much as I could, but the hemorrhage was very bad this time. I called his parents to come in and help. The doctor had suggested we wait for an hour to see if the bleeding stopped before going to the emergency room. An hour later it was still bleeding. I called the ambulance. I looked at the blood, then looked at Callum and wondered if he would make it through the night.

"Do you want me to call the kids?" I asked.

I didn't know what to expect or how to tell for sure if he was dying at home. I didn't want to overreact. I also didn't want to assume that everything was going to be fine. My hope was that he would get through it again. I looked at the fear in his face and heard the fear, and acceptance, in his voice. I knew I needed to be prepared for the worst. I didn't want to alarm the kids and call them to come so late at night for no good reason. The only fear bigger than Callum dying that night was the fear that I was in denial and wouldn't call the kids in time for them to say good-bye to their dad. From what I had read I learned that often the patient knows best so I decided to honour his wishes. It took a lot of pressure off of me.

"Yes. I think that would be a good idea. This might be the night."

Jamie and Vanessa got to the apartment before the ambulance arrived. I guessed with it being the fourth ambulance call in two weeks, we lost the priority status. We waited forty-five minutes for it to arrive.

That was the longest Callum had ever bled. We got to the emergency room and the doctor examined him. His vitals weren't great but weren't bad enough to be admitted. The doctor instructed him to keep pressure on the stoma to try and stop the bleeding. The doctor and I started talking about what had been happening the past two weeks.

"He won't even lay down to sleep anymore," I explained. "He sits up, with his hand covering his colostomy bag. He doesn't want to start bleeding and not wake up. I set my alarm for every hour through the night so that I can check on him."

I had no idea how bizarre that sounded until I saw the look of disbelief in the doctor's eyes. He was momentarily speechless.

"Are you connected with palliative home care?" he asked.

"Yes, we are," I answered.

"Have you mentioned to them that you are getting up every hour through the night to check on your husband?"

"No, I never thought of that."

I was so used to looking after everything myself I never thought of asking for help. It had been offered. I didn't think we were at the stage to need help. I didn't understand that this wasn't normal. I was used to

Callum's medical crises. I was used to doing whatever it took to look after him. I never considered that I could use some help.

Around 4:00 a.m. we returned home. The bleeding had stopped. There was time to catch a few hours of shuteye before I had to get up to take him for a blood transfusion. It was already scheduled and after that bleed, there was no doubt he needed it.

The next morning, Wednesday, we were having breakfast and the phone rang. It was the palliative home care nurse. She offered to have Callum stay a night in the hospital so that I could have some respite. He said he would go as long as I stayed with him. At first that seemed to defeat the purpose of me getting respite. Then I thought, at least in the hospital the nurses can check on him at night and I didn't have to worry. It also gave us more time alone together. He did know best. It may not have been perfect, but it was a step in the right direction.

When we were getting ready to leave that day, I had a sinking feeling. Honestly, it was a deep fear that Callum would not be coming home again. I remembered a couple of mornings recently he would wake up and say, "Well, I guess it didn't happen last night."

He had been eating less and bleeding more. He was more tired and weak. I had a hunch that once he was in the hospital he would decide to stay. Things had been getting less and less manageable for me.

I had decided to take him to the hospital in the Porsche. If, by chance, it was his last ride, I wanted it to be in his car. It was his pride and joy. I wanted him to have every possible ounce of happiness and enjoyment out of the Porsche. We arrived at the hospital and quickly got settled in. The room was quite small and easily got crowded when there was more than one visitor. It wasn't too long before he called to me.

"Lorna, I think I should just stay here for a few more days. One night isn't enough."

I knew this was coming. I knew he wasn't coming home.

"Maybe it will be just until Friday. I'm not sure, but a few days would be good. I want you to stay with me."

"OK." I said. "We can talk to the nurses about it. I don't know what we have to do, but they said you can stay here anytime you want."

Callum was admitted until at least Friday and was moved to a larger room. One immediate thing to sort out was what to do on Thursday, which was Cade's second birthday. We didn't want to have him die on Cade's birthday. The nurses and Dr. Foley were agreeable to help make sure he lived past then. It meant more blood transfusions, which would lead to more bleeds, but it was worth it. We made arrangements for Vanessa to have the birthday party in his room.

When Dr. Foley came to talk with us that day, he was up front and, at times, blunt. Callum was not doing well at all. The blood transfusions were helping very little. In fact, getting the extra blood was causing the extensive bleeds. It wasn't even staying in his body long enough to do any good, other than to keep him alive an extra day or two. Dr. Foley had a heart-to-heart discussion with us on prolonging life versus prolonging death. He agreed that there are cases where it is appropriate to prolong life, and sometimes those measures, in reality, prolong death. That he didn't agree with. That is what the blood transfusions were doing.

It was time to be realistic and get our priorities straight. We knew for sure we wanted to keep Callum alive until after Cade's birthday. That was goal number one, and we'd look at other decisions on Friday.

Thursday he had another bleed. It was getting more and more obvious that he was bleeding as fast as he was getting transfusions. Other than that, Thursday was an amazing day.

Vanessa brought an Elmo cake and cupcakes for the birthday party. Stuart's family joined us, and we had the celebration in Callum's hospital room. There were gifts all over and Cade rode his tricycle up and down the hall. We tried to respect the other patients and still give Callum the joy of celebrating Cade's second birthday. Considering we thought he might not see Cade be born, we were pretty ecstatic he was alive for birthday number two—even if we had to have it on a palliative care ward. Life is for living. So we did.

Thankfully, Stuart's mom was thinking and took a photo of our family. It was the last family photo we would have. I saw a picture of a family, full of love, sharing the joy of Cade's birthday. That picture means the world to me.

Friday morning came, Callum woke up, and with surprise said, "It didn't happen last night."

I couldn't imagine what it would be like waking up, wondering if I was still alive or in the next life. I certainly couldn't imagine what it would be like at night, closing my eyes, wondering if I would ever open them again. He didn't like talking about those things.

Another day. Another transfusion. Another bleed. That one scared the crap out of me. There was blood everywhere. All Callum wanted to do was pee. His mind was foggy, and he didn't understand why I was telling him to not stand up. I pushed the call button and the nurses came into the room in a flash. They had a lot of work to do so I left them to do whatever they needed to do. I didn't want to be in the way. I texted everyone I could think of and said they should come to the hospital. I was convinced he was going to die right then and there.

He cleaned up really well, and when I went back in the room I wouldn't have been able to tell that anything had happened. The nurses explained to me that they had packed his stoma so if he did bleed anymore, the packing would soak it up.

"How is he going to poop?" I asked.

The nurses stood there and stared at me. I looked back at them. They didn't have to say anything. I got the message. He was dying. There would be no more bowel movements. I was in such a state of shock you could have pushed me over with a feather. This was it. This was really it. Our days, maybe hours, together were numbered. It was time for another discussion with Dr. Foley.

"Well, Mr. Scott," Dr. Foley said. "We talked about getting you through your grandson's birthday and we did that. The transfusions are not doing any good anymore. They are only delaying the inevitable and causing you and your family stress. We have you scheduled for another transfusion this morning. I would suggest you not have it."

There it was again. That two by four of reality, slamming on my head and in my heart.

"If he doesn't have the transfusion, how long will he have?" I bravely inquired.

"It might be a day, maybe two. It's hard to say," Dr. Foley replied.

I turned and looked at Callum. His wish was that when he passed away our immediate family, his parents, and brothers would be with him.

"Do you want your brothers here now?" I asked.

"Yes. Yes, I do," Callum said, matter-of-factly.

"When would they get here?" asked Dr. Foley.

"It's a twelve-hour drive for one of them, so it might be a day or so, depending on how quickly they can get away," Callum replied.

"Well, Mr. Scott. Do you want one more transfusion? If it were up to me you wouldn't have another one, and we'd let nature take its course. Since you want your family here I am willing to go by your wishes with one more. But that's it."

"OK," Callum said, with resignation. "One more. Just so I can see my brothers one more time."

"Deal," Dr. Foley replied.

The conversation was almost too calm. It was hard for me to wrap my head around the fact that we were planning how to make him live long enough to see his brothers one more time. No tears. No shaky voice. Calm. I had moved into a state of acceptance. Or was it shock?

The following days were a blur. Not only did Callum not leave the hospital, I never left until he passed away. Surprisingly, it was quite nice staying there. There was a bathroom with a shower in his room so I could clean up every day. I had my own personal locker for my things. There was a love seat with reclining seats and a recliner chair for some comfortable seating. They were even good for naps. He wasn't eating so I was offered his hospital meals. Most of the time they were tasty. All of the time they were appreciated. Each night, they rolled in a cot and put it tight up against his bed. I slept better on that cot in the hospital than I had slept for months. Callum knew exactly what I needed.

I had read that when someone is close to dying, the nerves that give pain signals to the brain quit working. I had hoped this would happen for Callum. Of all the things he had gone through I wanted him to be relieved of the pain he felt in his knee. The bone had disintegrated so much from the cancer that the nerves were basically raw and rubbing together.

Unfortunately, it seemed like the pain intensified over those few days. I am not sure if it was part of his dying process, but I seemed to have kept better control of the pain at home. In the hospital, he had a self-administered morphine pump for pain control. When he was sleeping, we would diligently press it every fifteen minutes to try and alleviate any breakthrough pain. Dr. Foley even tried using a pain medication that was used for horses. It really didn't help. As the pain worsened, he would take more and more sedatives so that he wouldn't feel the pain. I yearned that he would be more alert so we could have more conversations. I couldn't stand to see him in such pain. I had to give up my wants so that he had relief.

Callum had many friends and the last few days he had visits from many of them. There was a sense of grace and respect mixed with immense pain during the visits. My heart broke each time someone would be in the room, holding his hand, telling him how much he meant to them, and they were going to miss him. It was tough to see grown men cry. It proved to me that he lived a great life. He was humble and surprised that he had made such a difference to people.

The hardest part for us as a family was to find a way to give these special friends the time that they needed to say good-bye without it interfering with our immediate family time with Callum. I was still dumbfounded and didn't really get it that the end was near. I might have appeared to get it. I might have even spoken like I got it. I didn't get it. I thought this would go on for days or weeks.

It would have been really helpful if someone had been blunt and said, "He is going to die in the next day or two. Do you really want friends and not family with him now?"

Looking back, I see now that the nurses really tried to give me the message. It never sunk in. I don't remember how many times they offered to put a sign on the door saying "immediate family only." His brothers and their wives arrived early Saturday morning. Finally, we started to block off time for the Scott family, and other times for our immediate family, Jamie, Vanessa, Stuart, Cade, and I. By this time, Callum was quite sedated to help with the pain from his knee. When he slept, we tried to sleep. There was comfort with us being together, even in silence. We were there for the few minutes he might wake up. We took turns clicking the dose of his morphine pump, sponging his lips, and holding his hand. There was no need to organize who would do what. It just happened.

Saturday night I felt a change and knew he was slipping away. Each night when I went to bed I held his hand until I fell asleep. That night he pulled his hand away. I reached further to hold it and he pulled it away again. The separation had begun.

Sunday was a quiet day. Callum was awake very little. We tried to feed him when he was awake but he refused. He was alert while friends had their brief visits in the morning, and slept most of the rest of the day. His brothers and parents spent part of the day visiting. I know he was comforted with being surrounded by the love of his family.

That night, Jamie and Vanessa had stayed with me in the room until late at night. We knew it wouldn't be very long and they were hesitant to leave. Jamie was giving Vanessa a ride home and he left to bring his car around to the front door of the hospital. Vanessa and I stayed in the room. Vanessa was on one side of the bed holding her dad's hand, and I was on the other side, holding the other hand. We tried to not cry. The tears just came. The sobs erupted.

Suddenly, Callum squeezed our hands and said, "It will be all right. It will be all right."

Those were the last words he spoke.

Monday morning came. Not much seemed to have changed. He continued to be heavily sedated and not communicative. He was slowly slipping away. We expected to lose him in the next day or so. He overcame so many challenges over the years that it was still difficult to really grasp that this was the end. I wasn't the only one who felt that way.

Vanessa had started a new job five weeks earlier. She wanted to show how responsible she was, so she went to work that morning. Her supervisors quickly got caught up on what she was working on and told her to go home. She was back at the hospital by 9:30 a.m. It was a good thing. Jamie, Callum's parents, and brothers were already there.

I sensed that he was hanging on for a reason. I was well aware that when people were dying, they sometimes needed final permission to leave. Callum and I had many talks about that moment. We had lots of time for him to say what he needed to say and to put things in place to make sure I was looked after. I thought we were complete. Perhaps he needed to hear it one more time.

I asked for some time alone with Callum. I picked up one of the small chairs, went around to the other side of the bed, put the chair next to his bed, and held his hand. There was no response. I looked at his face. He looked calm and serene.

"I love you so much. I know you love me, too."

Tears started to fill my eyes and my voice started to crack. I cleared my throat and started again.

"You have so many friends who care about you. You made a difference in their lives. They are thankful for the time they had with you."

I took his hand and held it tightly between my hands. "We had a great life together. We struggled and we had lots of fun times. I am grateful we never gave up on our marriage. I guess it's a good thing both of us were too stubborn to give in!" I said with a little giggle.

I carried on, more sombrely now.

"We have two wonderful kids. Jamie and Vanessa love you so much. You are a great dad. They are going to miss you. I am proud that you made your peace with them."

I sat for a moment while I collected my thoughts. My eyes filled with tears, I took a deep breath, and carried on. "Oh, and Cade. He is so lucky to have you for a granddad."

The tears rolled down my cheeks. First one, then two, then a stream down each side of my face. It was all I could do to control the sobs. "I know how much you love Cade, and how much you love being a granddad. We will make sure he never forgets you."

The sobs took control. I had to let them come out. There was so much heartache knowing my grandson, and the grandchildren to come, wouldn't have their granddad. I sat there for a few moments and cried.

I wiped the tears from my face, took a few more deep breaths, and continued.

"There are so many things we can be thankful for. Thirty-two years together. And to think most people didn't even think we'd stay together six months. We sure showed them!" I said with confidence.

"I will always remember special times like the weeks at the Tamarack Golf Tournament and taking the kids to Scotland. I loved our trips to Mexico. We saw a lot of great bands, didn't we?"

I knew it was a rhetorical question. I also knew that in his mind he was saying yes. I knew if he was more alert there would be a big grin on his face. I also knew he was preparing to go because there was no outward change in his expression to anything I said.

"Thank you for supporting me and for caring for me. You did a great job being the provider, and I am so lucky you agreed to be my husband. Thank you for believing in me and the things I wanted to do. I know it wasn't always easy to live with me and my crazy ideas. I am proud to be your wife."

The tears started flowing again. I choked through the tears and kept going.

"It's incredible, that with us so stubborn, we could find a way to become best friends. Your love and support made me a better person. I am going to miss you so much. The kids are going to miss you. I don't want you to worry anymore. I will be OK. Jamie, Vanessa, Stuart, and Cade will be OK."

I stood up, bent over the rail of the bed, gently kissed his lips. "Callum, it's OK to go. I am ready to let you find your peace. You fought a great battle as hard as you could and now it's time for you to rest." I bravely said through the tears.

"I love you, Callum. I always will," I said as I cried. "I will miss you forever."

I gently kissed his lips again.

We had asked for some immediate family time from 1:00 to 5:00 p.m. that day. With few changes happening it seemed like a safe thing to do. Vanessa, Jamie, and I took turns holding his hands, swabbing his lips and talking to him. The nurses came in, gave him a wash and a shave. I thought that was just their Monday job to do. I know now it was because they knew it was only hours before he would pass away.

About 3:00 p.m. I sensed something was different. I couldn't put my finger on it. I just knew it was time. I called the rest of the family back to the hospital.

When my dad died, I remember my mom saying, "It won't be long now." I hadn't noticed anything different and wondered how she knew. I didn't understand exactly how she knew. That afternoon I had learned that you just know. I hoped I could reach everyone Callum wanted to have there before he passed away. After days, months, even years of waiting, it would soon be over.

It didn't take long for the family to arrive. We offered any friends or family there a few minutes to say good-bye and then closed the room to immediate family, Callum's parents, and brothers. Again we took turns holding his hands, talking to him, and surrounding him with great family love. I was sure this would support him in his transition.

Around 5:30 p.m. Callum's breathing noticeably changed. We gave him our last kisses and each of us said, "I love you." As we joined hands to complete the circle of family love, the nurse came in and listened to his heart.

"He's gone," she said as his heart beat for the last time.

At 5:45 p.m., Monday, July 11, 2011, Callum passed away. His soul was gone. No more pain. No more cancer. He found peace.

The story of life is quicker than the wink of an eye,
the story of love is hello and goodbye...until we meet again.

~ Jimi Hendrix, American musician, singer and songwriter

REFLECTION

I now realize that I didn't have a clear mind in those last few weeks. At some point I should have found my own caregiver. I wasn't capable of making proper decisions. If I was to go through this again, I would have asked for more advice and more help. I would have definitely stopped our friends from visiting so much and for so long. I wish I had done that sooner. There was at least one day that he spent more time visiting friends than family. I wish I had listened to the nurses and put the "immediate family only" sign on the door. The best decision I made during that time was staying with him at the hospital. That is sacred time I will never forget.

TIPS

1. Have discussions with your loved one about where he/she wants to be when they pass away, who they want to have there, and any other requests they may have.
2. Pre-plan the funeral. Lots of details can be taken care of beforehand, and it ensures the wishes and desires of your loved one are honoured. There are enough things to be done afterward that pre-planning can lessen some of the stress.
3. Delegate someone to be your objective observer. This is a person who you can trust will tell you when you need help, and what you need help with. They can give you feedback on how you are coping and when you might need respite or other reinforcements. They can also look after your personal needs in those last few days.

TIME FOR YOUR REFLECTION

1. What are some of the conversations you need to have, and with whom?
2. What do you want your loved one to know before they pass away? Is there anything you need to tell them?
3. What does your loved one want in those final hours? Who do they want to have there? Do they want to be in the hospital or at home?

Chapter Eleven

Travelling Through Grief

Death leaves a heartache no one can heal,
love leaves a memory no one can steal.

~ *From a headstone in Ireland*

I'll never forgot the first time I experienced a great loss and found myself trying to grasp the mystery of grief.

On the morning of June 11, 1970, I was nine years old and busy getting ready for school. I heard a knock on the door and tried to take a quick peek out the window to see who it was.

"Stop looking out the window and get ready for school!" my mom emphatically urged me.

She went to the door and opened it to see a police officer standing on the other side.

"Are you Sheila Bodnaruk?" he asked.

"Yes," my mom replied.

"Do you have a son, Stephen James Bodnaruk?"

"Yes," my mom timidly replied.

"Mrs. Bodnaruk, I regret to inform you that your son, Stephen, died in a car accident last night. We need you to come and identify him."

Instantly, my mother burst into tears. I remember trying to figure out what was going on. My brother Stephen, twenty years old, had been away working and I seldom saw him. I didn't really grasp the seriousness of the situation. My mom called our neighbour and asked her to watch my brother and me while she went with the police officer. I knew something was horribly wrong when I was allowed to miss school that day. My nine year old brain and heart understood very little of the commotion.

Over the next days, weeks, months, and years, I was witness to how different people experienced and coped with grief. The day we found out that Stephen died was the first time I remember seeing my father cry. I saw how people were hurting so much they didn't know how to explain such a tragic accident to a nine-year-old girl. I was included in all the funeral rituals, though I didn't understand most of them. What I found the most difficult to handle during that time was watching so many people cry. Their pain and crying was contagious. I cried along with them. One vivid memory I have is the scent of our living room, full of beautiful floral arrangements from loving friends and family. For years, the smell of carnations and chrysanthemums reminded me of death, sadness, and grief. That symbolism was so strong I refused to have any of those flowers for years, including bouquets and flower arrangements for my wedding, nine years later.

That was just the beginning. By the time I was thirteen years old I was a funeral veteran. In March 1972, when I was eleven years old, my neighbours had a house fire and their two children, Robbie, aged four, and Angela, only one week old, died in the fire. Later that summer one of my friends, twelve years old, drowned while on her summer vacation. Within the next two years, another friend drowned and my grandfather passed away. I had lived through many tragedies, learning more and more about grief and loss. Now I realize that those experiences were fundamental in preparing me for the future. The knowledge and experience was helpful, but nothing could fully prepare me for how to cope with the profound loss when Callum passed away.

The experts in dealing with grief and loss highly recommended that a person make no major decisions in the first year following a major loss. That was one suggestion I didn't follow. Circumstances in my life immediately led to major decisions: selling our Saskatoon home and buying a new home in Medicine Hat. I didn't think I had much choice. The plan all along was to move to Medicine Hat permanently. With an insured mortgage on the house in Saskatoon, it was prudent to wait until he passed away before selling. Within a month of Callum's passing, I put the Saskatoon house up for sale, and a month later, I had sold that house and bought a new one in Medicine Hat. Looking back, I realize that I could have given myself more time to choose a house. I ended up selling that new house six months after I moved into it.

At the time, the reasons made sense. I had the itch to build a new house for more than five years. I knew the location where I wanted to build and the initial city development plan was that lots would be available in about two to three years. With the new home industry in Medicine Hat nearly stalled, and current developments far behind anticipated completion dates, I started to look at what was currently available. My sights were set on one of three or four lots. In early February 2012, just seven months after Callum died, I decided I should put a deposit on my favourite lot. I'd have up to three years to start construction and I could be patient about building. I was met with great disappointment as that lot was purchased only a few days earlier! All of a sudden, I was in a panicked state. I looked more closely, and seriously, at the remaining lots that were the right size and shape for the house I wanted to build, and in a budget I could afford. There was one left. With no idea how long it would take for new lots to become available in the next stage of development, I leaped a few years ahead of schedule and decided to build right away.

There was no doubt in my mind it was the best decision. I felt unsettled, both in the first house I bought and in the rental I lived in while I was building. The safety and security I felt in my new home was clearly evident days after I moved in. Then, I was finally able to express the deep grief I felt from losing Callum. That is when The Scream showed up. I had been plagued with feelings of anxiety and uncertainty while I was living in the duplex. I never felt really settled and kept myself quite guarded. The new house was my creation and it welcomed me. It was a symbol of the new me and made a perfect safety net for the release of grief. I could finally let my guard down.

The energy I used to keep my guard up was soon converted to energy required to expel grief. The tenseness in my muscles started to relax. I could feel it drain from my body. As it drained, the emotions started stirring in my stomach. First they brewed and then they erupted. The initial scream came from the depths of my body. Other times, there were unexpected outbursts of tears and sobs, over and over again. It would happen when I was writing the book. It would happen when I unpacked his personal things, like his watch and kilt. It would happen when I was alone in my bedroom. Sometimes I had to stamp my feet and pound my fists. It was uncomfortable at first. I was used to being the calm and rational one. But when the energy would boil and rise up, I had to do something. Especially when it started at the tips of my toes and travelled all the way to my head. I even had to throw things. I kept some control over that and chose soft things that wouldn't damage my new house. Stomping, pounding, and screaming were my go-to emotion releasers. Now I am more calm and at peace in my home. I am safe to be me. It has become my sanctuary. But it has taken time and I've faced many obstacles.

The long-term effects of stress and continually living on adrenaline rushes took its toll. I was an adrenaline junkie and didn't know how to stop or slow down. After Callum passed away, my body took over and forced me to slow down. For months, I couldn't make it through the day without taking a nap. I would sleep thirteen hours at night. I had no idea I was that fatigued.

I also noticed an inability to concentrate for really long periods of time. One time, when I was out shopping for houses with my sister Karen and brother-in-law Brent, I nearly rear ended a car and ran over a boulevard in the condo parking lot. I had driven in that lot for more than six months and knew it like the back of my hand. My thoughts couldn't keep up to my actions. When I was packing and unpacking during my move, I was easily distracted and would sometimes just sit there wondering what I was doing. I literally felt like I was thinking and moving in slow motion and didn't know how to speed up. There were times I was detached from myself, watching me from somewhere else. I saw myself wandering around like a lost child, not sure which direction to go first. I saw a woman, longing for life as it was with Callum. A woman trying to sort out what her next step would be as she entered a whole new world without him.

I knew the first year would be difficult to get through. Everyone talks about the firsts. For me, one of the firsts was just getting through the first month. The first night I spent in the apartment on my own was the hardest. I was fifty years old and, for the first time in my life, I lived alone. There were other times I was scared and anxious about being in unfamiliar territory: I was not sure I was ready to return to Saskatoon without him; something, or someone, was missing when I played with our grandson Cade. I remember one day I was so excited about something that happened to me, I rushed to the house to tell him, only to be abruptly reminded it was an empty house with no Callum, and no supper waiting on the table. I would have given anything to have him back.

Memories of the weeks and days before he passed away would flash through my mind. I saw him squeezing Cade's hand and smiling. I remembered when he held Vanessa's and my hands and said it was going to be all right. I remembered how Jamie lovingly held his hand for hours. I remembered listening to his breathing slow down, and when the nurse listened to his heart and said, "He's gone." He was finally at peace and pain free. And we were left heartbroken, with the task of carrying on our lives without him. I was not sure I knew how to do that.

A couple of weeks after Callum passed away, I received some information on grief and healing. There was proof that I was quite normal. But that didn't help. I wanted to move past the pain, but I read that it was necessary to move through the pain. The pain, when it showed up and how much it hurt, was beyond my control. I could only control how I handled those situations. I needed time to cry, be mad, eat well, exercise, be alone, and have fun. I needed to be around people, but have time to myself. I needed to have fun and have joy, but have days to mope, watch some movies, and temporarily hibernate. That was what was normal and expected.

It was the start of moving from "we" and "us" to "me" and "I." I emphasize start. It took me nearly two years to really stop saying "us," "we," and "ours." It still slips out every now and then. Which leads me to another point. How do you go from being a wife to being a widow? It is an interesting transition. I often wondered what was the first feeling people had when they heard the word "wife" and what was the first thing they thought of when they heard the word "widow?" "Widow" is a word that sounds so lonely and sad. And it is lonely and sad being a widow, especially when facing all those "firsts" without him.

The first big "first" was our wedding anniversary. I knew it was coming and kept myself busy as I prepared to move into my new house. Making arrangements for movers and cleaners kept me focused on the present, not what I was missing. I did what I thought was the "right" grieving and carried on. That would only work for so long. I could think I was in control of the grief. Yet, it took a life of its own.

September 29, 2011. Exactly one week past our thirty-second wedding anniversary. I was going along quite happily that day. I managed to get an eye exam on short notice and attended the Annual General Meeting of the Medicine Hat News Santa Claus Fund. I dropped off my Saskatoon phone modem, a huge bonus for me, as I didn't have to mail it back. I went home, grabbed a snack, had a great chat with a good friend, and started to do some unpacking. I decided to carry on with my bedroom and unpack the rest of my clothes. I opened the large brown wardrobe box from Saskatoon and took out a couple of my jackets. Next were Callum's clothes. I didn't have time to go through them in Saskatoon and brought them to Medicine Hat to deal with them. I hung them in the closet. I don't know why. At first it seemed like they belonged there. It made sense. Then it happened. I "hit the wall." My arms and legs had no strength. They felt like huge lead pipes. Almost like a paralysis. I was looking at things but not seeing them. I tried to make sense of my thoughts, but I couldn't. Intense fatigue and heaviness in my body was followed by cloudy thoughts.

It was a "hit me over the head with a two by four" cue that I was still grieving with some intensity. I felt that intense feeling only three times prior to that day. My first memory was the day Callum was diagnosed with rectal cancer. That foggy brain feeling of trying to make sense of what was happening. My second memory of that intense feeling was the day we found out the cancer had spread to both lungs and a cure was no longer in the picture. My third memory is of the day he nearly died from sepsis. The last few months I experienced a wave of these feelings, with varied intensities. But I was still taken aback that day with the suddenness of this wave.

I made it through the other "firsts": the first Christmas, his birthday, my birthday, Jamie's birthday, and Vanessa's birthday. I chose to have a celebration for the first anniversary of Callum's passing. *The Medicine Hat News*, where Callum's Alberta newspaper career began, bought a memorial bench that sits in the park behind the newspaper building. A gathering of family and friends celebrated Callum's life with a candle lighting ceremony and the unveiling of the bench. We enjoyed beef on a bun and visiting after the ceremony. I look back and see that being busy, organizing all of this, was my coping mechanism. It was something for me to focus on, so I didn't have to pay attention to what was really going on with me.

It is what I have always done. Ever since Callum was diagnosed with cancer, and maybe even before that, if something was hard to deal with, I got busy. The anniversary of his transition from this world would be no different.

I put the focus on him. We missed him. We loved him. We wanted to honour the life he lived, and the life he gave us. It was a good excuse for me to not show how much pain I was in. No one would have to know how many sleepless nights I'd had. Or how often I could still smell him, see him and hear him. Of how much my heart ached every time I saw the family and friends "couples" and realized I no longer was part of a "couple." The crowd that surrounded me, in love and support, would know nothing of how alone I felt. It was a celebration of Callum's life and a good place to focus. It helped me hide the pain.

The bench unveiling and memorial service helped me get through the day. It did little to help me heal from the grief.

What surprised me was how hard the second year was. I think I was so prepared for the first year that I assumed the second year would be a cakewalk.

What was very odd to me was that the hardest days were Valentine's Day and my birthday. We didn't even used to make a big deal about Valentine's Day. That was the weird part. Yet, leading up to that second Valentine's Day, I was filled with anger and resentment. I thought it was all fake. All these lovey dovey couples. They weren't truly in love, were they? It all came down to the fact that I was alone. The world around me was focused on couples.

I was overcome with sadness when I woke up alone on my birthday. There were small thoughts that I was being selfish. I missed the "Happy Birthday" and a hug first thing in the morning. It was hard to have that for over thirty years and then not have it. I missed the anticipation of where we would go for supper, and what gift he bought. I loved my birthday, the time spent together, and the gifts. I never made it a secret how much I loved gifts!

I wouldn't have made it through the first few months without the support of my counsellor, Gail. It was mandatory that I seek counselling as long as I was on disability payments. That was a good thing. Gail listened to whatever was going on for me at the time, provided information, and tools to deal with the emotions, and helped me gain insight into some of the things that were happening, and how I was feeling. I didn't want to burden family, who were dealing with their own grief. Newly returned to Medicine Hat, I hadn't re-established many close friends in whom I could confide. The friends who were close were also dealing with their own grief from

Callum's death. A counsellor was the perfect option to get over the first hump. A deeper benefit was having someone who was objective, was very familiar with grief, and the grief process, and had my best interests at heart.

My massage therapist was another important member of my healing team. Her keen sense of intuition helped her tap into whatever was the priority for healing that day. She shared her spirituality and empowered me with new healing techniques. She always knew exactly what I needed. One of the first times I went for a treatment, she spent about ten minutes just rocking me like a baby. I hadn't realized how little touch I had in those first few months after Callum passed away. It was not a typical thing you would expect when going for a massage. It was just what I needed for healing at that time. We have grown to become friends, and I am very grateful she is in my life.

To round out the team, I brought on Lisa, my personal trainer. I knew from past experience I wasn't ready to commit to going out of the house to exercise. I was referred to Lisa, and thought that if she showed up at my house, I would have no option but to exercise. It was a good plan. For nearly two years, she regularly came to my home and put me through the paces. In the summer of 2013 we had some scheduling conflicts, and it became more difficult to continue with our sessions. She was a very important part of my healing from grief. After years of neglecting my body, the regular exercise helped me increase my strength and stamina. Most importantly, it gave me a physical outlet to express and release the anger, frustration, and sadness from the grief I was feeling.

Slowing Down

One of the arduous things I had to become aware of, and deal with, was the drive to do everything possible in a three-month time frame. I didn't fully appreciate how much that was a habit until I over-scheduled myself and kept saying "yes" immediately to things/events that could wait a few more months, or years. I had to learn to trust that there would be other opportunities to take a course or vacation. When Callum was alive, we had to grab onto every opportunity when it came up. I rearranged my work schedule, and we moved around treatment schedules so Callum could experience as much of life as possible. It didn't matter to me that I worked evenings or weekends to make that happen. It didn't matter to me that I worked when we were at the cancer centre or visiting in Medicine Hat. It didn't matter to me that we went into debt to make as many of Callum's dreams as possible come true. For over a year after his death, I continued the mindset that there wasn't going to be a tomorrow. As my energy was challenged and my bank balance decreased, I took a look around at everyday people doing everyday things, and realized it was time to change my thoughts. It was time to move from impulsivity and into more strategic planning. It was time for me to go after my dreams. I now had time to do it.

Whenever there was a bumpy course in my life, I fought back. I intentionally sought out positive and inspirational outlets to get me back on track. I remember back in the mid-1990s after my "best boss ever" left the YWCA Westman Women's Shelter to take another job. Morale decreased, other friends left, and soon it was a place where I felt unhappy. Then I discovered *Chicken Soup for the Soul* by Jack Canfield and Mark Victor Hansen. The wonderful collection of inspirational short stories gave me the attitude change I needed. I soon had a different outlook on life, which helped me take the action needed to change jobs.

That was my first introduction to Jack Canfield. I was enamoured with the *Chicken Soup for the Soul* series and continued to buy many of the new books. Then came *The Secret* by Rhonda Byrne. There was Jack Canfield again, this time talking about the law of attraction. The idea that we get to create our own thoughts, and therefore our own life, was intriguing to me. And it was free to try, so I went ahead and tried. I followed Jack Canfield on his website and listened to the monthly "Ask Jack" calls whenever I could. In 2009, when he started his Train the Trainer program, I longed to be part of it. The obstacle in my way was the three weeks of live training that was held in the United States. With Callum's fight with terminal cancer, I could not afford to take time off to do such an intensive training program. I had little energy and an uncertain financial future, so the dream was buried.

Over the years, I found many tricks to stay in joy and happiness when things in my life appeared miserable. I would look for uplifting success stories, inspirational quotes, and things that made me laugh. During one rough period at work I even subscribed to Joke of the Day email. At least I knew I would have one laugh that day. I found a "pot of gold" full of inspiration on the Internet. I subscribed to Notes from the Universe, a service of TUT.com (Totally Unique Thoughts). Monday through Friday, "The Universe" would send me an inspirational message. That would be the first thing I would read in the morning and it would set the tone for a positive day. During another particularly difficult time at work, I started collecting happy faces and covered my office in them. I had a cell phone stand, magnets, candy bowl, coffee mug, pictures, candles, night-light. Anything I could find with a happy face found its place in my office. There were so many that when a new staff person took a tour of the office building she asked if I loved Wal-Mart!

Six months after Callum passed away, I knew I needed to move through the grief and intentionally wanted to help the process along. The Canfield Training Group was promoting its Breakthrough to Success program. The week-long personal development training took place just after the one-year anniversary of his passing. I wanted to find the new me. Really, it was the old me who needed to be rediscovered. My intention was to be released of the anchor of grief, loss, and guilt that still enveloped me.

I felt so guilty that I was alive. I felt so guilty that I had the financial resources to go to the Breakthrough to Success course. I didn't believe I deserved to have the life I was living. I'd give it all away if Callum would come back. I knew that could never happen, and I still had to find a way to release the hurt, guilt, and anger. It was time to do what worked in the past. I wanted to find a way to process those feelings in a healthy and positive way. Jack Canfield and the *Chicken Soup for the Soul* books years ago had helped me. I'd listened to his monthly call for a few years now. I was looking for a breakthrough. It was staring me in the face. Breakthrough to Success 2012. It was just what I needed.

Looking back, I realize the guilt started to incubate the moment we found out the cancer had spread and Callum had terminal cancer. When I think back to that moment, I can remember saying to myself, How am I going to make it without him? Which was quickly replaced with: It's not fair that he's going to die. How can I worry about me when he's dying?

That was it. The seed of guilt was planted. Over the next three years it would be fertilized, watered, and nurtured. It kept me humble. It stole my power.

I had no regrets that Callum became the centre of my universe. I truly believed that it was my mission, and passion, to help him live the best life he could for as long as he could. That is how guilt works. It took something honest, compassionate, and sincere, and twisted it around so that I would feel guilty for things I couldn't control.

The week spent at Breakthrough to Success, with Jack Canfield and 340 other wonderful people, was a phenomenal first step. When the week was finished, I looked around the room and saw people, from doctors to former homeless people, who made huge changes in their lives because of Jack and The Success Principles. The book alone helped one man go from being homeless to being a successful entrepreneur in less than two years.

I had been helping people for years. I believed in this positive, solution focused method and having a chance to learn from an expert had me hooked. I had been waiting for over three and a half years. I signed on the dotted line and applied to take the 2013 Train the Trainer program with the Canfield Training Group. Little did I know at the time that it was a huge leap to becoming "me."

I approached my journey through grief like I approached most things in my life. I attacked it. I researched it. I called on others to help me. I found positive inspiration through stories, other people, and looked for ways to process the hurt and the pain. All the pieces fit together like a puzzle. The counselling, massage, reading, writing, and sharing with other widows all kept me moving through the grief. The personal work I did during the time I spent training with Jack Canfield released a lot of the pain and gave me strength to keep going. I was introduced to a mind/body technique designed to heal emotional wounds and dissolve self-sabotaging beliefs. The RIM® Method—Releasing Your Inner Magician— was created by Dr. Deb Sandella. This healing modality accelerated my journey through grief and really helped me move from "we" to "me." I was blessed to find Kathy Sparrow, a writing coach who is also a Master RIM® facilitator. Writing about my story has been one of the most important things I have ever done. It has also been one of the most emotional things I have endured. Working with Kathy not only helped me write a great book, she was also there to help me through the roadblocks I faced while writing. This two-pronged approach to my book was instrumental in the transition I made so far. My journey through the grief puzzle was pretty complete.

Not Everyone Heals at the Same Pace

I've been told that everybody experiences grief differently. That each one of us will move through the grief process in our own time. When Callum died, I don't really remember thinking about that at all. I knew people were hurting. I thought they hurt like I did. It wasn't a conscious thought, but I assumed they would deal with the loss in the same way I did. Or at least find their way to deal with it. I stayed in my bubble I created when he was sick. I didn't look outside myself. I do remember looking at my children, wondering how they were doing. I was concerned about them and hoped they had someone to talk to. I hoped they would seek counselling if they were finding things too tough to deal with. That was as much effort as I could put into other people at the time. I was temporarily done looking after others.

Looking back, I realized that not everyone around me had all this knowledge, or the tools, to deal with their grief exactly like I did. My issues were not their issues. Everyone experienced their own loss and had attachments to different parts of Callum's life. My eyes were opened to how different this was on two occasions, both over two years after he passed away.

During the trip to Scotland to scatter Callum's ashes, my sister-in-law, Dorothy, asked to speak to me, alone. I noticed everyone at the table get up to leave and didn't think much of it.

"I have to ask you something. It's been bugging me for a long time and Alan said I should ask. Why wouldn't you let me be in the room when he died? What did I ever do to you, or him?" she asked, her voice shaking and tears rolling down her cheeks.

I was shocked. I was certainly not expecting that question.

"I didn't make that decision. Callum did. I didn't ask why," I replied. "He was dying!" I exclaimed. "I can't explain his thoughts. I might have made a different choice, but that was his decision. I just honoured his wishes."

"Well, that makes it worse because I can't even ask him," she cried.

"I am sorry," I gently replied. "That decision was about him. It wasn't about you."

"Well, it hurt me. I think it might have hurt Linda too, and that's why they have been a bit on the cold side."

I was at a loss to say any more. I didn't have an answer. Those last few days Callum was in the hospital were a blur to me. There was no energy or brain power to rationally discuss or question anything that was happening. If he had asked me to shave my head and paint my body orange, I would have done it. That is the state I was in. What other people thought was no consequence to me. Callum was the only one that mattered.

Dorothy's question saddened me. For over two years, people in my family had been hurting over this. It had affected our relationships. My image of our tight-knit family was suddenly shattered. I couldn't help but wonder what else had upset people. I had no interest in having to explain or justify myself. My only desire was to get the issues out in the open and resolve them.

For more than two years I knew something was wrong, and I badly reacted to the discourse, oftentimes judging other people in my family. My mistake was not asking earlier what was going on. I could have saved us months—even years—of frustration and sadness.

Surprise number two. It took only a few seconds after Jamie arrived at my house for me to realize this was an intervention a few weeks in the making. He and Vanessa had been having very deep, intense, and emotional discussion about their concerns before coming to see me. They were worried about two things: my financial situation and my health.

We differed on our perspectives of how to handle each situation. There was misinformation, which fuelled their worry and concern, and their emotional outburst.

They were passionately concerned that if I didn't get control over my health that they would lose another parent at too young an age. They were most concerned about my health. I had been overweight for years and they worried I would die young and they would have no parents. I couldn't fault them for that. They had lost their dad at too young an age. They didn't want to be without the one parent they had left. They didn't know that I had continued working with a trainer for exercise and was taking Isagenix® supplements to assist in keeping up with the nutritional needs of my body. Having my dog, Pepper, pretty much guaranteed I'd be out each day walking. What was missing was a true deep down commitment by me.

Jamie and Vanessa asked that I take on a healthier lifestyle, weight loss, and exercise with as much enthusiasm as I do the rest of my life. During the Canfield 2013 Train the Trainer program, I noticed nearly everyone in the group really valued their body and treated it well. I learned from that and decided it was time for me to take charge of my life, lose some weight, and get into better shape. If I was going to live the life of my dreams I would need all the energy I could possibly get. The plea of my children would not go on deaf ears.

The more delicate subject of finances was brought to my attention. Jamie and Vanessa were carrying out Callum's wishes for me and really wanted to make sure I had every opportunity to build my business and live my dream. They offered, in no uncertain terms, their perspectives and suggestions on what they thought I needed to change to make this happen. The missing piece to their puzzle was that I had a mind of my own. I knew what I wanted. I went after it. I didn't take the exact path that Callum had thought I should take.

They heard I had considered selling the Porsche. Unknown to me, this was devastating news to them. So much so that Jamie said he wouldn't speak to me if I sold the car. I knew it was something special to own a Porsche, even if it was thirteen years old. Yet, I often felt awkward when I drove it, wanting to apologize for having it. I felt guilty that the only reason I had the car was because he died. I wasn't the proud Porsche owner that Callum was. He really loved the Porsche. It was something extremely special to him. I loved the Porsche. It had different meaning to me. I felt little attachment to it. I suspected that might change if I ever did seriously consider selling it.

"Mom," Vanessa explained. "That car was a symbol of the hard work Dad and you did in your lives. How you proved you could be successful even though everyone told you that you'd never make it."

I finally understood. That was their attachment to the Porsche. I knew why selling the Porsche was such a volatile subject. For me, it was the Toyota Avalon that was the symbol of his hard work. We bought the Avalon after moving to Red Deer. It was luxury we had never known. He was on the rise in the newspaper industry and the Avalon was the symbol of that status. I had already practiced saying good-bye to those symbols. I personally watched, and joined Callum, in the grief of losing the Avalon, the tangible symbol of years and years of work and sacrifice. I was there when he said good-bye to his staff, and to his career. I had cried and been angry. I had grieved that loss. Five years ago. I'd had time to process and overcome it. I had come a long way since then. To me, the Porsche was a symbol of a bucket list item. It was a car for Callum to have because he was dying. I saw it as a symbol of a life cut short.

During his illness, I had moment after moment of saying good-bye to these important symbols and started grieving their loss before he passed away. I was determined to not to be consumed by more grief any longer than I had to. I couldn't control the fact that my husband was dying and I was going to be a widow. I supposed I couldn't really control how fast I worked through my grief. I could, though, use the knowledge, skills, and tools I had to help me heal from losing my husband, and come out on the other side joyfully living the life I have left.

At first, I was disappointed at their outburst, spurting out inaccurate information and combining all their concerns into one big giant mess. Of all the people in my life, I counted on them to stick up for me. It took me a few days to realize they were. It sure didn't come out that way to me at the time. I realized they were really coming from a place of grief and fear. They couldn't understand where I was coming from because they weren't living my life. They were clinging to their dad's final wishes. As they should. They didn't want to disappoint him. They didn't want me to disappoint him.

What I realized was that once again, we were on a shared journey, yet each of us also walked it alone. Jamie, Vanessa, and I had been worried so much about comforting and protecting each other during that time that we didn't want to burden each other with our grief. We talked about Callum. We'd tell each other how much we missed him. Only once do I remember actually saying anything about how our lives were different without him.

"It's not fair," Vanessa whined. "Since Dad died I don't have anyone left who thinks like me. You two and I don't think the same." She was addressing both Jamie and me.

"What do you mean?" Jamie replied. "I miss Dad because I don't have him to help me see things the way he would see them. I now have only one person who thinks differently than me."

The relationships Callum had with others affected their personal grief journey. It affected what we would hold on to and what mattered most to us about him, our relationships, our memories, and what symbolized all of that for us.

I knew too well that life doesn't go exactly as we want it to. Callum had dreams for me. They were based on the best information we had at the time. Two years later my dreams were based on new information and decisions I made. The worst thing I could do for me was to continue to live in the past. It had taken me more than two years and a lot of work to start to discover who I was and learn how to make it on my own. Things changed. I knew deep in my heart that Callum's biggest wish was that I do what I love to do. That was what I was doing.

He was gone. I was here. It was time for them to shift from "we" to "me."

Not until we are lost do we begin to understand ourselves.

~ Henry David Thoreau, American author and poet

REFLECTION

The fact I had been a counsellor and aware of grief and loss issues helped me through some tough times. It came with a cost, though. It kept me on the intellectual side of grief and didn't allow me to deal with the emotional collateral from Callum's passing. I thought I could overcome anything. I thought I was strong. That was until I was forced to deal with my own grief. I learned that grief was hard to figure out. It was often disguised as sadness, anger, or guilt. It was there one minute and gone the next. Well, more accurately, it wasn't there, and all of a sudden it showed up in the strangest places at the strangest times. It would pop up while I was sitting outside, while at a band concert, or while driving. There was no telling when the tears would well up, when waves of heaviness would invade my body, and my mind would come to a screeching halt. But I made it through.

TIPS

1. Create your support team. Some people to consider:
    a. Grief counsellor
    b. Grief support group
    c. Massage Therapist
    d. Yoga Instructor
    e. Personal trainer
    f. A good friend
    g. Financial advisor
    h. Medical doctor
2. Talk with your family, especially your immediate family. Be honest about your feelings about missing your loved one and the impact it has personally on you. Most likely everyone shares your thoughts and feelings. Include some time to talk about how you can support each other through this time.
3. Give yourself plenty of time to rest, physically, emotionally and spiritually. Don't make any major decisions in the first year. If you are forced to make a major decision, enlist some experts to help you.

TIME FOR YOUR REFLECTION

1. What are some of the other experiences you have had with grief, and what did you learn?
2. Describe what things you miss about your loved one.
3. What are five things you wish people knew about what you are going through, and how can they help you?

Chapter Twelve

Epilogue

All the art of living lies in a fine mingling of letting go and holding on.

~ Havelock Ellis, British psychologist and writer

It was a miracle that day, Sunday, September 22, 2013. The sun shone brightly against the sapphire blue sky and sent warmth not yet felt since I arrived in Scotland. Three days earlier, the wind was cold enough for Jamie to wear a toque (knitted cap) when we were looking for the perfect place to scatter the ashes. I had told Callum that since it was his ashes we were scattering, the least he could do was help us out with good weather. He lovingly obliged.

I thought this day would never come. When he passed away two years earlier, I felt a sense of urgency to honour his wishes of being returned to the North Sea, near his birthplace. However, the years leading up to his death wore all of us out. Vanessa was expecting a baby, and all of the family had taken enormous amounts of time away from work before he passed. We were ready for a break. I was ready to rest. It didn't take long to decide we would delay the trip to Scotland until 2013. So much had happened since then.

Callum was a popular guy and built many close business relationships and friendships in both Brandon and Medicine Hat. I knew these friends and colleagues would want a chance to say good-bye and honour Callum, so I planned memorial services in both cities. Both services were living proof of what great a man he was, and his life well lived. I thought after the first it would be easier to do the second. I was wrong. It was even more difficult to say good-bye a second time.

The final good-bye lay ahead of us, and I was determined to keep my promise to him. He left some decisions up to me and the ones he made were deeply important to him. And so they became deeply important to me. I would have gone anywhere he asked to have his ashes spread. It made sense to me that he returned to where his life began. Callum would have thought about this for a long time and his request would have come straight from his heart. Everyone in the family knew this.

Family was the most important thing to Callum. It took me a number of years to gain insight to the depths of his love and admiration for his family. I knew he would love to have as many family members in Scotland as possible, even though he accepted it might be only me who would be able to go. With his spirit as my guide, I invited our families to join me in taking him home. It was a precious time to be joined by our children, Jamie, Vanessa, and Stuart; Callum's parents, Mary and Walter; and his brother Alan and Alan's wife, Dorothy. His brother Glenn and family had other family priorities and were not able to come with us. I was excited that my nephew and his wife planned to be with us. Sadly, they were affected by record flooding in our city and had to cancel their plans.

I like harmony and peace. I try to take into account everyone's wishes and desires and this trip was no exception. Ironically, my drive to have harmony and peace brought discord and frustration! Any attempt at coordinating schedules for ten people turned out to be an exercise in futility. And when we thought we had it all worked out, the flood hit and key players in my plan were no longer part of the package. I had planned to travel with Chris and Raegan on September 15th and we were going to hang out together in Edinburgh. Between a little sightseeing, some shopping, and golf, we had three days on our own. Stuart and Vanessa would meet up with us three days later. It was such a great plan—until Mother Nature became involved. Little could be done about the devastation Chris and Raegan faced with flood damage. It was no longer possible for them to make the trip. So my plans changed.

I travelled alone. Well, I did carry Callum with me. Before I left on the trip, I wondered how many awkward moments I might have taking an urn of ashes over to Scotland. It didn't take long before I encountered the first uncomfortable conversation.

I juggled my luggage and the urn, discovering how heavy ashes were! One of the best mistakes I made was having my jacket on top of the bag with the urn in it, and forgetting to check it in with my other bag. It would have cost me an extra hundred dollars in excess baggage fees to take him!

As I made my way to security, I told the officer that I had an urn of ashes. The line came to a screeching halt. The urn could not go in any ordinary plastic tub. Oh no. The security officer called for a special plastic tub. The bottom was grey foam, about three inches thick. There was an indent running down the middle of the foam so the urn could lay down and not roll. Here I was, lugging my carry on, purse, and urn. And who got the special treatment? He did!

Once again, pushing and pulling the various pieces of luggage, I finally arrived at the desk of the United Kingdom Customs in Scotland.

"Hello," she said, expressionless. "How are you?"

"I'm fine," I answered. I don't say any more than necessary when going through customs.

"Are you travelling alone?"

"Yes, I am."

"What is the nature of your travel?" she asked. Again, no expression.

"I'm here to visit family," I replied.

I didn't want to get into a long drawn out conversation trying to explain everything. I thought I could keep it simple.

"And what family do you have in Scotland?"

Busted. Clearly, I was not Scottish. It was time for a little backpedalling.

"Actually, it's my husband's family I am visiting."

It had to happen.

"And where is your husband?" she asked, not missing a beat.

It seemed like an eternity for me to gather my thoughts. I had a quick peek at the bag in my arms, the bag holding the urn. A number of quick comebacks ran through my brain. Thankfully, common sense took over.

"My husband passed away and I have come back to scatter his ashes."

"Oh, I see," she said, still with no expression.

I watched as her hand reached for the custom stamp. She grabbed the stamp and with a bang, my passport was stamped and I was clear to go.

"Welcome to Scotland," she murmured as I put my passport away for safekeeping.

Since I was travelling on my own, I decided to start the trek to Fraserburgh. My son, Jamie, was arriving the next day in Aberdeen, only forty-five minutes from Fraserburgh, our final stop. After a frantic few hours on the Internet and phone looking for a reasonably priced place to stay, I settled on taking the train from Edinburgh to Dundee and stayed the night.

There was no doubt I had foreigner written all over me. There I was, a lady, all alone—a large suitcase in one hand, a smaller carry-on bag in the other. Somehow, I balanced my purse and the urn, too. I wonder if I was on any TV top ten laughs of the day! This was a time I really missed Callum. Four hands and shoulders were always better than two. I got it down to a science and managed to pull and push all of it at the same time. I walked out of the Edinburgh airport to find the bus that took me to the train terminal.

It was an adventure. I got on the bus to the train station and rushed to catch the next train that was leaving in eight minutes. As I pulled two suitcases and lugged a purse and an urn full of ashes, I had flashes of temptation to leave the urn of ashes in Dundee. Would Callum have really ever known? The comedy continued.

I made it to the train on time. Barely. I was so grateful for the gentleman who offered to help me store my luggage. My cases were quite awkward for getting through the narrow aisles on the train. A jiggle here and a jiggle there and I was set. I was happy to have a few minutes of rest.

I got off the train in Dundee. It was a little station, so inside the building it was easy to find the signs to the taxi stand. They pointed up the stairs. I looked up the flight of stairs and took a big gulp. My eyes scanned the other signs in the building. Intense relief came when I found the sign for the elevator. I had no clue how I would have made the stairs with the pile of luggage I was crating along with me.

My excellent adventure was not yet over. The taxi driver started loading my cases into the trunk of his car. I let go of my carry-on bag and instantly it tipped over. The black handle made a beeline for the passenger side door. I looked up to see a thick black mark, about six inches long, that was a stark contrast to the shiny clean white door. I was sickened. I didn't want to spend my first day in Scotland dealing with trying to figure out what responsibility I had for the damage to the car. It was starting to feel like this was not going to be an easy trip in any way, shape, or form.

Luckily, after about fifteen minutes of elbow grease, cleaner, and a shammy, the taxi driver was able to remove the black mark. Another moment of deep gratitude. The worst thing that happened was that I was a few minutes late to the bed and breakfast, arriving about 2:05 p.m., five minutes past the deadline for the early check in. I had let them know that I may be later than 2:00 p.m. and hoped someone would still be around to let me in. It had been nearly twenty-four hours since I left home to start the trip. I was ready to be settled for a few hours.

The taxi driver helped me get the luggage up the stairs to the front door of the guest house. I knocked on the door. A stern lady opened the door. The look on her face would have scared off a U.S. Marine!

"Hi. I'm Lorna," I said with a smile. I was hoping my good Canadian kindness might warm up the frozen personality standing in front of me.

She rolled her eyes at me. "Lorna? Lorna who?" she demanded.

I suppose it was my false expectation that after a few emails and booking and paying for my room that I thought they would be expecting me, and would know my name, at least my first name. The woman just never warmed up. I pulled all my gear through the double doors, thankful to be in one place for the night.

"You know your room is on the third floor, right?" she said, with a high degree of arrogance, as she took a long look at the suitcases.

"Well, I didn't know that. I guess I will make as many trips as needed to get everything upstairs," I replied.

I had nothing else to say. I had prepaid the room and had no desire to try and find somewhere else to stay. By that time, I was used to having some kind of challenge to whatever I faced that day. Three trips later, I was settled in my room. I unpacked only what I needed for the night, went down the road for supper, and was in bed by 7:00 p.m. I was scheduled for the 8:30 a.m. breakfast sitting and a good eleven or twelve hour sleep was in order.

I woke the next morning feeling grateful for a good night sleep and more gratitude that I was there for only one night. I had breakfast, showered, packed, and had a taxi called for me. I was looking forward to a smoother day. I'd meet Jamie, Auntie Beryl, and Uncle John, and get settled in my new home for the next week.

Outside the B&B, the taxi driver lifted the cases, and I could tell by his expression that he was surprised at the heaviness as he picked up the smaller one. "What have you got in there, a dead body?" he said with a laugh.

Awkward moment number two. The urn was now in that suitcase. I couldn't help but laugh like crazy on the inside. I had to quickly decide what to say.

"Well, sort of." I replied. "I'm here to scatter my husband's ashes and his urn is in there."

That was quite the conversation starter. I figured he'd either be embarrassed, and it would be a quiet and peaceful ride to the train station, or else he'd appreciate the humour and we'd have a wonderful conversation. It was the latter and I quite enjoyed the Dundee history lesson during the short ride to the train station.

The rest of the day went smooth and my timing couldn't have been better. I arrived at the Aberdeen train station, which was next to the bus terminal. I walked up to the information window and asked where and when to get the next bus to the airport, where I was meeting Jamie, Auntie Beryl, and Uncle John. Five minutes later I was on my way, and arrived with plenty of time for lunch before Jamie's flight landed. Perhaps things were changing.

I found Auntie Beryl and Uncle John, and after Jamie got his luggage, we were on to the next leg of our journey. We were Fraserburgh bound! I was looking forward to catching up with the Scotland family. Things work out the way they should. I was disappointed to not have the three days in Edinburgh with Chris and Raegan. However, I realized that these days were now a gift for me to have time to relax and get everything ready for the scattering ceremony on Sunday.

It seemed like it should have been an easy thing to organize the scattering of ashes. I needed a time, a place, some people, and somewhere to mingle afterwards. The time was chosen first. Some people were travelling, so mid-afternoon seemed like a good time. That was set. Sunday, September 22, at 2:00 p.m. we planned to gather to say our final farewell to Callum. With the "when" looked after, it was time to find the "where."

On Wednesday, Jamie and I started the search for the perfect spot. Callum loved the shore near his cousin's house where I was staying, and that was the first place we looked. The spot was beautiful and I knew why he loved it. It was a very rocky shore, and it would have been quite a walk out to the water. His parents wanted to spread some ashes, and I knew they would never make it down the rocks to the water. Beautiful place. Not practical.

We continued down the shoreline. The wind was quite chilly and reminded us to keep in mind that it could be raining on Sunday. We needed to find somewhere that wasn't going to be muddy or slippery when wet. This started to become a challenge. We walked up and down the shoreline. Everything seemed to be a steep angle down to the water, or so rocky it was tricky maneuvering, even when dry. Some of the local family suggested the old lighthouse on the pier. As we were coming near it, we thought it would be a nice place. We got near the pier only to find out that due to some wicked storms, the lighthouse was being repaired and the pier was closed. That day's hunt for the perfect place came to an end.

The next day, Kerry, our cousin's daughter, took me to look at some more places. We went to the stream near the golf course. It was absolutely beautiful and looked like a perfect setting for a scattering ashes ceremony. There were a few little hills and I was worried about the condition the shale path would be in if it rained. Right near the water was a bit soggy and I wasn't sure it would withstand all the people standing on it. The final straw was that it wasn't really the North Sea. It was a creek that ran into the North Sea. On we went.

We checked out the beach. Kerry had mentioned there was a bridge right on the walkway and then we might not even have to go onto the beach. However, the bridge had been wiped out and the best trail closed, likely due to the bad storms.

I was starting to feel like I was the fussiest person in the whole world. I just wanted to make it easy for everyone, young and old. As a last resort, we headed to the pier by the shipyards. It was perfect. When we looked out over the sea, it was never-ending. The pier was made of cement and so large that people could park on it. Only a few steps would be necessary. There were three different directions we could scatter the ashes, depending on the wind direction that day. My heart instantly felt warm, and I felt so calm and peaceful I knew this was the place.

The big decision was out of the way. I had already arranged for family to gather at the Fraserburgh Golf Club following the ceremony. That would be the only time that I would have to visit with some of them. The golf course was perfect because there was lots of room and we wouldn't have to hurry. I didn't want to put anyone out by expecting them to open their home up to twenty-five or thirty people. I was happy things were falling into place.

Jamie and I did some visiting, and we started to let people know the final plans for scattering the ashes. It seemed like this day would never arrive and now it was upon us. I wasn't so busy anymore now that the plans were completed. Reality started to set in, and I wondered if I was really ready to let him go. It was a bizarre thought that my mind tried to accommodate. After more than two years since Callum passed away, I wondered why it seemed hard to let him go.

Saturday, September 21. It was the night before scattering the ashes. The most bizarre, most unbelievable, and most comforting thing happened that night. I had come to love Twitter and noticed my great-niece talking about a new app. It sounded cool, so I tried to download the SnapChat app to my phone. That was when the surreal happened. I was supposed to reply to a text message to confirm the app download. What showed up in that text feed astounded my children and me. Somehow, in one of the text messages I received while doing this, was Yoda's quote on death:

"Death is a natural part of life. Rejoice for those around you who transform into the Force. Mourn them do not. Miss them do not. Attachment leads to jealousy. The shadow of greed that is."

I have no idea how this happened. What made it that much more surreal is that Callum and I both loved Star Wars. We used to joke with him that his personal higher power was Yoda and his funeral would be a Star Wars theme. In the deepest, most delicate part of my heart, I knew it was Callum sending me a message.

However, even that couldn't wash away the anxiety and sadness that had been creeping into my being more and more each day—and was beginning to overwhelm me. Thursday was the first time I let myself admit this was more than a ceremony. It was the final farewell. I began to wonder if I was going to be able to follow through with it. An image instantly popped into my mind. It was of me, holding the urn, guarding the urn, not letting anyone take him. Until then, I hadn't realized I was so attached to the cremains. I thought I had moved on.

The feelings that were so strong at the memorial services started to return. It seemed cruel to put my children through this again. We were just getting back to being a normal family. Once again, I wondered whose wishes were most important? We all wanted to respect Callum's wishes. He wanted his ashes scattered here. This was the third time, wait, the fourth time we were saying good-bye. Talk about pulling off the Band-Aid® slowly. I really hoped it was going to be easier. Deep down I knew it likely wouldn't.

All was in place. The short ceremony was planned and would be followed by a toast to Callum, and visiting. It became more apparent in each passing minute that it was going to be a tough day. That night I could feel the tears start to flow. I prayed for strength. It was time to let him rest and for me to have the final parting. That was hard to think of, particularly as I filled ten little boxes with ashes for anyone who wanted to personally scatter some. I packed a small cardboard box with the urn, the little boxes, some red wine for the toast for anyone who didn't like Scotch, a corkscrew, an extra sweater, and my camera. There were quite a lot of things for a simple ceremony.

I knew this was weighing heavily on me, and my energy. I looked forward to completing something left undone for over two years, freeing up energy that had been protecting me from feeling for so long. There would be no telling which emotions would show up. The relief of the final farewell, mixed with the sadness of saying good-bye, would be a defining moment for me. Life does go on.

Slowly, I opened my eyes and saw the morning sun peek through the bedroom blinds. It was the first clue that it was time to rise and shine. This was going to be the day. The final good-bye to my love, Callum. The overwhelming feelings of wanting to take the urn and run away dissipated and were replaced by feelings of sadness, a little anger, peace, and hope.

I made my way to the kitchen and put the kettle on to make coffee. I sat down at the table and opened the patio door. The sunshine pouring through the doors was a welcome sight. I could hear the chirping of birds and knew we would have a great day. I had asked Callum to give us a nice day, and he lovingly obliged.

In the summer of 2012 we had a family meeting to plan this very special trip. We took into consideration work schedules and responsibilities, personal commitments, and preferred time of year to travel. With ten of us in the mix and all considerations taken, September 22 was the chosen day. With no pre-determination planned at all, we were to scatter Callum's ashes on what would have been our thirty-fourth wedding anniversary. I felt too young to be a widow, and certainly too young to have been married thirty-four years ago.

As the time to leave approached, each of us got our best clothes on and we were ready when Allison and Uncle Alistair arrived to pick us up. We drove onto the pier and could see that some family had already arrived. The weather was beautiful and, in fact, it was the best weather of the entire trip. The beautiful blue sky was a colourful backdrop for the bright yellow sun. Only one or two wispy white clouds were visible, and there was hardly a breath of wind. It was warm enough to not need my extra sweater.

The family arrived. We exchanged hugs and kisses. Everyone milled around taking in the breath-taking weather. We thought it would be quiet on the pier on a Sunday afternoon. Two groups of fishermen tried their best to continue fishing. Once our group of thirty was in place, Caroline, a girlfriend to our cousin's son, played the bagpipes before the ceremony—a very special treat for us. She gave a big squeeze to the bag as the sweet sounds of "The Flower of Scotland" reverently surrounded us. Thankfully, the fishermen decided to take a break and give us space. We had the pier to ourselves.

I placed the urn on the cement wall on the pier. The wall was about three and a half feet high and a foot wide. Jamie lined up the ten boxes with the ashes on the ground in the centre of the circle. They would be ready and available for anyone who wanted to spread ashes.

I stood there, soaking up the love and support of our family. I looked at the paper with the ceremony written on it. I was ready.

"Thank you …" I started.

In an instant, my hands began to shake, tears filled my eyes, and I started to choke on the words I was trying to say. The tears ran down my cheeks. I felt the sobs form in my chest and rise up to my throat, where they collided with the words I was trying to say, effectively choking them off. I thought I was ready. In that moment, I had to question myself on that thought. I have to get through this, I said to myself. You can do it. You can do it. You can cry later. Get it together for the next few minutes. I took a few deep breaths, wiped my eyes, cleared my throat, and continued.

"Thank you for joining us today. We are so grateful that all of you have come to give Callum a final farewell."

I started to feel more calm and settled. The words on the paper helped provide focus for me and I was brought back to the present moment. Jamie came and stood next to me, his arm across my shoulders. The next few moments were filled with inspiration and a celebration of Callum and his love for family, and his life. After a brief moment of silence, Caroline once again played the bagpipes while we scattered Callum's ashes. Love, sadness, relief, joy, peace, and hope were palpable. I walked over to the middle of the circle, bent down, picked up a gold box of ashes, turned around, and walked to the cement wall. I stretched over it as much as possible, said to myself, You are home, Callum. Rest in peace. I love you, and let the ashes dance through the air, softly falling on the water.

One by one, Jamie, Vanessa, Stu, Walter, Mary, Alan, Dorothy, and other family members walked to the middle of the circle, picked up a gold box of ashes, walked to the edge of the wall, opened the box, bent over the wall, and lovingly sent Callum home in the North Sea.

Mary, Callum's mother, walked over to hug me. Tears flowed freely down her face. We gave each a squeeze of love as we hugged.

"It isn't any easier two years later," she whispered in my ear.

Alan, Callum's brother, brought the group back together again. Plastic shot glasses were handed out to everyone, followed by the sharing of a bottle of Scotch and red wine. Alan shared his special memories of his brother and a life well lived.

"Please raise your glasses in a toast to Callum," Alan said.

"To Callum," the group cheered.

Hearing those words made my heart fill with pride and contentment. I could rest knowing he had a good life and he was finally at home.

The whole service and toast took less than twenty minutes. There was time for everyone to have their own moment of silence, thoughts, and reflection about Callum. The sea was so calm that day. Everything was perfect.

Mary came back over to me. She pointed to a church steeple just up the hill from the harbour.

"Do you see that steeple?" she asked.

"Yes, I do." I quizzically replied.

"Just to the left of that steeple is where we lived when we brought Callum home from the hospital. We used to put him in his car bed right by the window overlooking this harbour."

Waves of emotion overcame me. Tears filled my eyes. I put my arm around Mary and pulled her close. This was news to me. I chose the harbour only because it was easily accessible for everyone. There had to be some divine guidance when I was looking for the perfect place to scatter the ashes. Something, or someone, guided me to the place where Callum's life began. His life had come full circle. Everything was absolutely perfect.

"He's really home," I said, as the tears rolled down my cheeks.

It was done. As promised, we returned Callum home. It was where he wanted to be. We gathered at the golf course to spend some time with family, visiting and enjoyed a meal. I was relieved it was over. I was surprised at how exhausted I suddenly felt. I wanted to visit with as many people as possible, especially those I wouldn't see again on my trip. It took a lot of encouraging self-talk for me to muster the energy to work my way around the table and engage in conversations. Everything was fine. I could go to bed early if I wanted. The last of the adrenaline oozed from my body and my lead-like legs carried me back to the house.

The next day, I realized my memory of the ceremony was slightly hazy. After all this time I expected to be in control and able to handle this last responsibility. I realized what happened. For what I hoped would be the last time, the shield of armour showed up when my emotions started to spill over, and the robot army was what gave me the focus to read the paper and carry on. Both of them protected my heart, my emotions, and the pain that came with the finality of the moment. That protection blocked some of the memories.

She was no longer wrestling with the grief, but could sit down with it as a lasting companion and make it a sharer in her thoughts.

~George Eliot, English novelist and journalist

Later that week, I flew to Portugal to visit with friends for a few days. It was a wonderful distraction from the emotional purpose of the trip. On the last night I was in Europe, I went out for supper. As I sipped on a tasty glass of red wine, I realized I was going home. Without Callum. I had focused so much on being faithful to his wishes, I hadn't thought what this moment would be like. There would be no more ashes in the urn. No more planning the trip to Scotland to scatter the ashes. I felt very melancholy. I wondered what life would now be like. He was part of my life, part of me, for over thirty years. An ocean once again would lie between us. A perfect symbol that it was time to leave him at peace, and for me to live my life.

The separation was final. No longer a "we." It was now time to live my life as me.

RESOURCE LIST

BOOKS

Janet Bray Atwood and Chris Atwood. *The Passion Test, The Effortless Path to Discovering Your Life's Purpose.* New York: Plume Publishing (a division of Penquin Publishers), 2007.

Canfield, Jack. *The Success Principles: How to Get From Where You Are to Where You Want to Be.* New York: HarpersCollins Publishers Ltd, 2007.

Hickmam, Martha Whitmore. *Healing after Loss, Daily Meditations for Working Through Grief.* New York: HarperCollins Publishers Ltd, 1994.

James, John H. and Russell Friedmann. *The Grief Recovery Handbook, 20th Anniversary Expanded Edition, The Action Program for Moving Beyond Death, Divorce, and other Losses.* New York: HarperCollins Publishers Ltd, 2009.

Levine, Peter A. *Waking the Tiger, Healing Trauma.* Berkely: North Atlantic Books, 1997.

Pausch, Randy. *The Last Lecture*, 2008. New York: Hyperion Publishing, 2008.

WEBSITES

CAREGIVER SUPPORT

Canadian Caregiver Coalition - www.ccc-ccan.ca

Caregiving.com - www.caregiving.com

Lotsa Helping Hands - www.lotsahelpinghands.com

PALLIATIVE CARE SUPPORT

Canadian Virtual Hospice www.virtualhospice.ca

National Hospice and Palliative Care Association - www.nhpco.org

GRIEF SUPPORT

Centre for Loss and Life Transition (Dr. Alan Wolfelt) www.centerforloss.com

The Centre for the Grief Journey - www.griefjourney.com

GENERAL CANCER AND COLORECTAL CANCER SUPPORT

Canadian Cancer Society - www.cancer.ca

American Cancer Society -www.cancer.org

Colon Cancer Canada - www.coloncancercanada.ca

ORGANIZATIONS

Colorectal Cancer Association of Canada - www.colorectal-cancer.ca

LIVESTRONG Foundation - www.LIVESTRONG.org

Imerman Angels - www.imermanangels.org

GENERAL AND LOCAL RESOURCES

The resources listed below are available in most communities, or nearby communities. Each location will offer their own unique support in the areas of visiting the family, providing respite, financial assistance, spiritual and emotional support and much more.

Look in your yellow pages or do an Internet search to see what is available in your area.

Faith-based institutions: Churches, Temples, Mosques

Service Organizations: Legion, Rotary Club, Lion's Club, Kinsmen, Kinettes, Optimist Club

Family Service Organizations

Social Work departments at the hospital or Cancer Centre

Counsellors and Psychologists

MeetUp Groups

Caregiver Coaches

Local Cancer Agency office

Local office for your disease/illness: Persons with Disabilities, Alzheimer's,

Multiple Sclerosis, Parkinson's Disease

Support groups for caregivers/patients

Corporations and Agencies

Charities and Foundations

WISH GRANTING ORGANIZATIONS

Canada

Canadian Wish Foundation
www.terriowen.ca

Ph. 416 699 2195 Toll free - 1 800 000 0000

Sunshine Foundation of Canada (for children)
www.sunshine.ca

Ph: 519-642-0990 Toll-Free 1-800-461-7936

Cleaning for Cancer Patients
www.cleaningforcancerpatients.ca

Ph. 905-633-7778

International

Starlight
www.starlight.org.uk

Adult Wishes Foundation
www.adultwishes.org

Cleaning For a Reason
www.cleaningforareason.org

United States

Air Charity Network
www.aircharitynetwork.org Ph. 1 (800) 549-9980

Dream Foundation
www.dreamfoundation.com Ph. (310) 444-3070

Second Wind Dreams
www.secondwind.org Ph. (678) 624-0500

The Angel Foundation
www.theangelfoundation.net Ph. (419) 238-6726

Unity, A Journey of Hope
www.unityajourneyofhope.org Ph. (724) 677-4789

Jeremy Bloom's Wish of a Lifetime
www.seniorwish.org Ph. (720) 889-2029

The Granted Wish Foundation
www.grantedwish.org

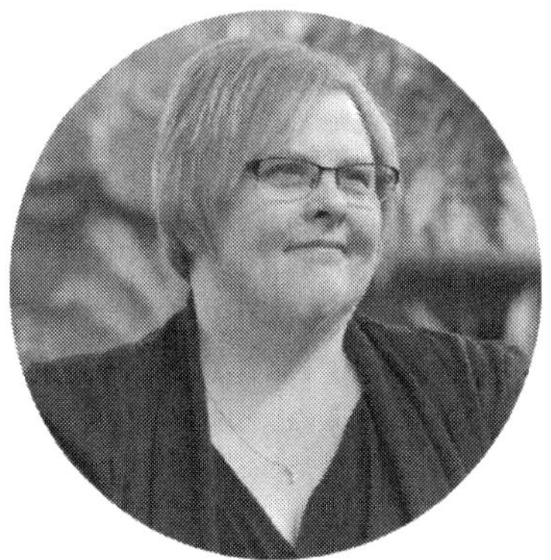

About the Author

Lorna M. Scott is the founder and owner of Accelerated Success Consulting. With over twenty-five years experience working in the human services field she found her passion helping others discover their own inner power and special gifts. During her personal transition and transformation following the death of her husband, she became passionate about the plight of the caregiver.

Lorna works with people who are ready to transform their lives, have more joy and live with passion. She is a trainer, self-development coach, author and speaker who has worked with individuals and facilitated groups for over twenty years. Her personal philosophy is to have a positive outlook on life with a focus on solutions, not problems. She firmly believes that with the right information, attitude, focus and a belief in yourself you can achieve your highest goals. Lorna passionately believes that these are the keys to unlocking your success and greatest gifts as a caregiver.

She is a graduate of a year long intensive and professional Canfield Training Group Train the Trainer Program, based on the book *The Success Principles*, by Jack Canfield. She is a Certified Passion Test Facilitator, a Certified Facilitator for Advanced Solutions for Activating Passionate Engagement, and an Opposite Strengths Executive Coach.

Lorna resides in Medicine Hat, Alberta, Canada, where she enjoys hanging out with her dog, Pepper, spending time with her son, daughter and their families, including three amazing grandchildren. She adds balance to her life by enjoying Toastmasters, golfing, and playing her flute in the community concert band.

Lorna's Keynotes

Lorna has been public speaking and sharing stories for many years. Her vast experience of working with people has built a solid foundation for captivating a crowd with her uplifting message of peace, hope, and joy. Many are inspired, empowered, and motivated by her message and leave feeling they have the power to change their life.

Lorna shares the trials and tribulations that she experienced as a caregiver—juggling the demands of a terminally ill husband, her children's needs, and her career responsibilities. Sprinkled with humour, she speaks of the valuable lessons she learned, particularly those on giving herself a little bit of her own attention and learning to ask for help. Allowing her audiences to peak behind the curtains of her personal transformation since Callum's passing, she shows us how she became a woman who is comfortable with living her life as "me" rather than "we."

Topics

"I Didn't Order This—Can I Send it Back?"

How to overcome the overwhelm of your new role of caregiver.

"Staying Strong: How to Look After You"

Find the strength and courage to look after you so you can be better at looking after others.

"Stop the Madness"

Key steps for creating a caregiving life with peace, hope, and joy.

Other Programs

Caregiving Mastermind Group

A mastermind group is a peer group of four to six members who support and challenge each other to create and implement goals, brainstorm ideas, and support each other with total honesty, respect and compassion. Who are the experts to help caregivers? Most of the time, it is other caregivers. A mastermind group of caregivers brings together the expertise of their experience and a venue to share their wisdom, receive guidance and support.

For more information go to www.walkingthejourneytogetheralone.com or Contact Lorna: E. lorna@lornamscott.com P. 1-403-548-8437

Caregiver's Coaching

Being a caregiver brings a wide variety of challenges. Many frustrations arise when trying to balance work, family, home—all while caring for yourself and for your loved one. Add to that the worry and concern about the future and how that impacts you, your loved one, family, and friends. Our systems can easily go on overload, and life can be an emotional quagmire. Let me help you find peace, hope, and joy in the journey.

For more information on how coaching will help you find more peace, joy and hope in your life, contact Lorna at:

E. lorna@lornamscott.com P. 1-403-548-8437

www.walkingthejourneytogetheralone.com

Made in the USA
Charleston, SC
02 September 2014